THE BLOOD HANDBOOK

```
H53585      COLL: 07/02/92 UNKNOWN  REC: 07/02/92 11:02 PHYS: ULTMANN, JOHN

    COMPLETE BLOOD COUNT
      WBC                    4.0     [3.5-11]     K/UL              STAT
      RBC                    4.89    [3.88-5.26]  M/UL              STAT
      HEMOGLOBIN             13.8    [11.5-15.5]  G/DL              STAT
      HEMATOCRIT             40.2    [36-47]      %                 STAT
      MCV                    82.1    [81-99]      FL                STAT
      MCH                    28.2    [26-33]      PG                STAT
      MCHC                   34.3    [32-35]      G/DL              STAT

    DIFFERENTIAL
      NEUTROPHILS            63      [38-77]      %
      BANDS                  0       [0-6]        %
      LYMPHOCYTES            30      [12-56]      %
      MONOCYTES              7       [1-15]       %
      EOSINOPHILS            0       [0-7]        %
      BASOPHILS              0       [0-2]        %
      REACTIVE LYMPHS        0                    %
      METAMYELOCYTE          0       [0-0]        %
      MYELOCYTE              0       [0-0]        %
      PROMYELOCYTE           0       [0-0]        %
      BLASTS                 0       [0-0]        %
      PLATELET ESTIMATION    ADEQUATE
      RBC COMMENTS           NORMAL
      ABSOLUTE BLASTS        0       [<0.1]       K/UL
      ABSOLUTE PROMYELOCYT   0       [<0.1]       K/UL
      ABSOLUTE BASOPHILS     0       [0-0.22]     K/UL
      ABSOLUTE EOSINOPHILS   0       [0-0.48]     K/UL
      ABSOLUTE MYELOCYTE     0       [<0.1]       K/UL
      ABSOLUTE METAMYELO     0       [<0.1]       K/UL
      ABSOLUTE BANDS         0       [0-0.66]     K/UL
      ABSOLUTE NEUTROPHILS   2.52    [1.33-8.47]  K/UL
      ABSOLUTE LYMPHOCYTES   1.20    [0.42-4.00]  K/UL
      ABSOLUTE MONOCYTES     .28     [0.035-1.65] K/UL
      ABSOLUTE REACT.LYMPH   0                    K/UL

    ESR, WESTERGREN          *21     [0-20]       MM/HR

    PLATELET COUNT           229     [150-450]    K/UL              STAT

    THYROTROPIN              ASSAY TWICE/WEEK WITH RESULTS TUE, FRI

    TRIIODOTHYRONINE         ASSAY TWICE/WEEK WITH RESULTS MON, WED

    THYROXINE                ASSAY COMPLETED DAY FOLLOWING RECEIPT

    UA CHEMSCREEN
      APPEARANCE             YELLOW
                             SLIGHTLY TURBID
                             TURBID
      SPECIFIC GRAVITY       1.022   [1.016-1.022]
                             TEST PERFORMED ON REFRACTOMETER. GLUCOSE
                                MOLECULE MEASURED.
      PH                     5.0     [5-9]
      URINE LEUK.ESTERASE    *POSITIVE
      URINE NITRITE          NEGATIVE
      PROTEIN                *TRACE
                             PROTEIN SCREEN IS INSENSITIVE TO GLOBULINS.
      BLOOD                  *3+     [NEG]
      GLUCOSE                NEGATIVE
      REDUC.SUBST.           TEST NOT PERFORMED   %
      KETONES                NEGATIVE
      BILIRUBIN              NEGATIVE
      UROBILINOGEN           0.2     [0.1-1]      G/DL

    UA MICROSCOPIC
      RBC                    OCCASIONAL           /HPF
      WBC                    5 TO 10              /HPF
      CASTS                  OCCASIONAL           /LPF
                             HYALINE
      EPITHELIAL CELLS       MANY                 /HPF
                             SQUAMOUS
      ORGANISMS              MODERATE
                             BACTERIA
      CRYSTALS               NONE
      OTHER                  MUCOUS THREADS
```

A typical printout of a lab report on a blood test

GEORG HOFFMANN, MD

THE

BRENDT BIRKNER, MD

BLOOD

EDITED BY

HANDBOOK

JOHN E. ULTMANN, MD

Hartley & Marks
PUBLISHERS

Published simultaneously
in the USA and Canada by:

Hartley & Marks, Publishers
79 Tyee Drive, Point Roberts WA 98281
3661 West Broadway, Vancouver, BC V6R 2B8

Printed in the USA

Text and illustrations © 1991
by BLV Verlagsgesellschaft mbH (München)
English translation © 1992 by Hartley & Marks, Inc.
See also p. 198 for further credits.

Originally published in German as
Das Blut—Steckbrief unserer Gesundheit
German text by B.R. Birkner, MD and G. Hoffmann, MD
Translated by Andreas Kahre
Translation edited by J.E. Ultmann, MD

ISBN 0-88179-084-2

If not available at your local bookstore, this book may
be ordered from the publisher. Send the cover price plus two dollars
for shipping to either of the above addresses.

LIBRARY OF CONGRESS CATALOGING-IN-PUBLICATION DATA
Birkner, B. (Brendt R.). 1948–
The Blood Handbook: a guide to blood tests in health & illness
/ by B. Birkner, G. Hoffmann : edited by J.E. Ultmann : [translated
by Andreas Kahre].
p.   cm.
Translation of: Das Blut.
Includes index
ISBN 0-88179-084-2 : $11.95
1. Blood—Analysis. 2. Blood—Examination. 3. Blood—Popular
works.
I. Hoffman, G. (Georg), 1954–   . II. Title.
RB45.B46   1992
616.07'561—dc20   92-34865
CIP

NOTE
The ideas, methods and suggestions in this book
are not intended as a substitute for
consultation with a physician.

TABLE OF CONTENTS

ACKNOWLEDGMENTS

I wish to acknowledge the diligent assistance of three of my colleagues at the University of Chicago Pritzker School of Medicine: Dr. Joseph M. Baron, MD, Associate Professor of Medicine, for his overall general assistance with the book, Dr. Monique Jacques, MD, Senior Resident in Pathology, for verifying the information in the Appendix, and Dr. Roger Stupp, MD, Fellow in Hematology/Oncology, for reading the German version and advising on points of clarification.

John E. Ultmann, MD
Medical Editor

FOREWORD

"Blood is a very special juice," Mephisto's famous words, have acquired a whole new meaning for modern medicine, because blood test results are now an indispensable part of nearly a third of all diagnoses. Patients are often confronted with lab printouts that are riddled with technical terms and figures, and that are unintelligible without detailed explanation. Abbreviations like GPT, T3 and T4, AFP and CEA contain the diagnostic building blocks that indicate to the physician liver damage due to alcohol, thyroid disease, or cancer. And often the meaning of these terms and how they relate to a complaint remain unclear for the patient—sometimes because the physician may not have enough time to offer an explanation, sometimes because the explanation needs to be more detailed, or more comprehensive.

In this book we offer interested readers the means to recognize the main connections between laboratory tests and various diseases, and to help them become informed patients, so that they can, with their physician's guidance, better maintain their health and fight against disease.

This book should help its reader recognize and understand laboratory test results like the ones we have included. We thought it important to not only list those diseases that can be recognized via blood tests, but to discuss their causes and relationships to the function of our whole organism, and to raise awareness of the risks of premature self-diagnosis.

Of course, the few chapters of this book cannot begin to replace the physician's medical training and the many years of clinical experience. But we hope they will, in a meaningful way, answer the questions that always arise during blood testing. This book contains the accumulation of years of clinical experience. It has been written with the intention of integrating both traditional medical knowledge and the more recent diagnostic methods and trends in laboratory medicine.

B. Birkner, MD
G. Hoffmann, MD

I

BLOOD IS A VERY
SPECIAL JUICE

B lood has always stimulated people's imagination. "Blood is a very special juice" are the words that Goethe, the German poet, puts into the mouth of Mephistopheles as the latter urges Faust to sign the devil's pact. In Europe Heart's blood was once poetically linked with the "ink" of love poetry and of farewell notes, and today a wealth of expressions demonstrate the symbolic power of blood: your blood may boil, or run cold, or you might have blue blood, but be unable to get blood out of a stone, all the same. Many of our expressions gain a theatrical or even ominous quality when they are connected with the image of blood.

In this book we examine the subject in a more sober way. Our blood is indeed a "very special juice," and one of the most important subjects of analysis in modern medicine. No tissue and no other body fluid has been studied more closely, and few medical techniques permit deeper insights into the functions and dysfunctions of the human organism than the microscopic and biochemical analysis of a person's blood.

Entire fields of medical specialization deal exclusively or primarily with blood—foremost among them being hematology (from the Greek *haima:* blood, and *logos:* word, science, thus "the science of blood"). Hematology, a subdiscipline of internal medicine, is the science of diseases of the blood, whose best-known examples are anemia and leukemia (cancer of the blood).

However, hematologic tests account for only a small portion of blood examinations. Blood cannot be understood in isolation. It flows through our entire body, it supplies all of our organs, disposes of their waste products, and it reflects our state of health just as a river reflects the condition of the environment through which it passes. That is why an area of specialization has developed based on general medicine, pathology, chemistry, biochemistry, and microbiology which attempts to discover the diseases of the blood itself and to supply information about the health of the entire organism. This is the discipline of laboratory medicine (lab medicine), which, as part of clinical pathology includes clinical chemistry, bacteriology, immunology, and hematology. This young discipline has established itself as an independent field of medical specialization only during the second half of this century.

Due to the rapid pace at which the natural sciences are developing, today's laboratory medicine is one of the most technologically advanced medical specialties. It plays a more and more important role in medical diagnosis and in monitoring therapeutic measures— identifying diseases and controlling the success of treatment. The average hospital processes several thousand blood samples each day, while some large laboratories process tens of thousands of such samples. Approximately one third of all medical decisions are influenced by or determined by laboratory test results—a highly efficient technique when one considers that the cost of blood testing in hospitals accounts for less than five percent of the total budget. Nearly every field of medical specialization involves the interpretation of laboratory test results, in particular the areas of general medicine, internal medicine, and intensive care medicine.

Without aspiring to the scientific detail of a medical textbook, this book is meant to offer a range of useful information from all of these areas, presented in an easy to follow format. It was conceived as a handbook for the medically interested among the general public, and as a guide for those who would like to find out more about the meaning of their own blood test results.

▸▸ Our Blood As An Organ

Nobody doubts that the liver, heart, and kidneys are organs. But the claim that our blood is also an organ may not convince you as easily. A liquid organ—a surprising thought at first.

Our everyday use of the word "organ" involves a variety of contexts, ranging from "organs of the press" to "organic economic growth." The term stems from the Greek *organon* and means generally *tool*. In medicine, our organs are considered as "tools of the body"—body parts with clearly defined boundaries and biological functions. That the blood fulfills certain functions is obvious. But where are its clearly defined boundaries? Doesn't blood appear throughout the body?

The boundaries of blood, our liquid organ, are defined by the walls of the vascular system. Blood streams through the arteries away from the heart into the capillaries and through the veins back to the heart. In medieval times and even at the beginning of the enlightened age it was believed that blood flowed only in the veins while the arteries conveyed air. This false conclusion was arrived at because in every autopsy all the blood was found clotted in the veins. Propelled by the pressure of the final heartbeats it just cleared arteries and capillaries before coagulating and coming to rest in the veins as a black-red mass. It was only in 1628 that the British anatomist Sir William Harvey published his, at that time, revolutionary theory of blood circulation. It was proven conclusively by the microscopic examinations of Marcello Malpighi, an Italian born in the same year as Harvey.

▶ *The Blood's Varied Functions*

The functions of the blood vary greatly and are based on its presence throughout the body. While single-cell organisms such as bacteria can carry out all vital functions, such as transporting nutrients, movement, reproduction, and defensive immune reactions, multi-cell organisms have cell types which specialize in particular responsibilities: muscle cells provide movement, nerve cells transmit signals, and liver cells carry out metabolic functions. The blood's tasks are mainly related to transportation, communication, and defense.

Blood provides transportation primarily for the oxygen which is essential for our cells' energy production, but all nutrients, waste products, salts, and hormones also use the bloodstream as a means of transportation.

Communication or "signalling" between our cells and organs is served indirectly by the blood circulation. All along the blood's "highway" stands a series of "weigh stations,"—organs with biological sensors which monitor physical and chemical properties of the blood, such as blood pressure, blood sugar level, or salinity. When needed they inject chemical signals into the blood in the form of hor-

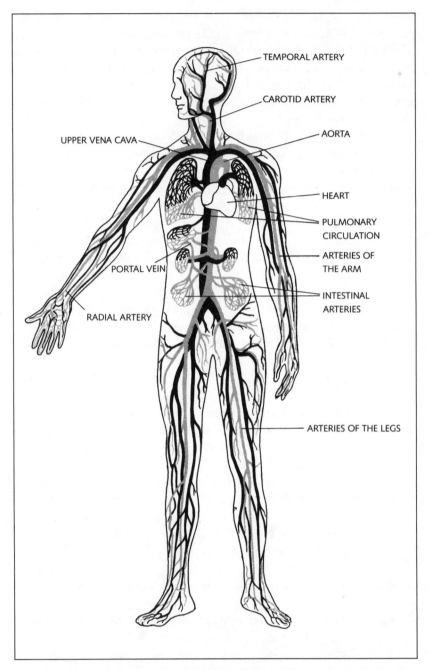

TEMPORAL ARTERY

CAROTID ARTERY

AORTA

UPPER VENA CAVA

HEART

PULMONARY
CIRCULATION

ARTERIES OF
THE ARM

PORTAL VEIN

INTESTINAL
ARTERIES

RADIAL ARTERY

ARTERIES OF THE LEGS

Our vascular system consists of arteries and veins, almost all of which run in parallel. (Not shown are the capillary blood vessels.)

mones or hormone-like substances, and in this way send "messages" to distant organs in our body.

Defending our organism against harmful substances, both from outside and within our body is the blood's exclusive and immediate task. Specialized phagocytes and leukocytes—the "white corpuscles"—continually probe every cell and every chemical substance in the body, and attempt to remove anything foreign and harmful.

It is not unusual for our organism to use one organ for a variety of tasks if they can be sensibly combined "under one roof." Thus, our brain is used not only for thinking, but also to regulate vital processes such as breathing and circulation. Our liver produces numerous vitally important substances, and at the same time filters their catabolic products (the substances that result from their chemical metabolic breakdown). Our pancreas helps with digestion, and also maintains a constant blood sugar level.

Our blood plays a similar role. As a liquid it is the only organ that can reach almost every corner of our body (except the cornea of our eyes, and the fluid encasing our brain). And that is why transportation, communication, and defense are concentrated in the blood. An additional task which our blood fulfills is to guarantee the integrity of the blood circulation itself. The coagulation process is used to identify injuries of the blood vessels within seconds and to seal them within minutes. When we consider all these functions it becomes clear that our blood really is an organ, and a body part with definite boundaries and clearly defined functions.

SUMMARY

Our blood, just like our heart and kidneys, is an organ of our body with definite boundaries and clearly defined biological functions. Its boundaries are defined by the walls of the circulatory system which can be subdivided into veins and arteries. Its functions are primarily to transport nutrients and metabolic products. It also serves as a means of communication among our body's organs, and works to defend us against harmful substances both from outside and within the body. The coagulatory system helps to protect the blood's circulation with blood clots to seal "leaks" in the walls of blood vessels.

►► *Our Circulatory System*

A grown man has approximately 9.5 pints (4.5 liters) of blood, women and children have a little less. By weight, therefore, our blood comes fourth after our musculature, fat tissue, skeleton, and before such important organs as our liver, heart, and brain. Our heart keeps the circulatory system moving by beating on average 80 times a minute, each beat propelling about .15 pints (.07 liters) of blood from the left ventricle into the body's main artery, the aorta. It takes only a minute, therefore, to pump our entire blood volume of more than four liters through the heart.

Without the elasticity of the walls of our blood vessels, the heart would not be able to maintain a constant flow of blood throughout the entire body. Instead, the blood would be accelerated with a sudden jolt with every heartbeat and would come to a sudden stop with the closing of the heart valves. This would lead to extreme pressure peaks during the acceleration phase and complete pressure loss during deceleration. Moreover, with every heartbeat, strong turbulences would form in the bloodstream and these could damage the blood vessels and blood cells.

In order to "smooth" these shock waves, our blood vessels are elastic, like rubber hoses, and expand with every heartbeat. During the heart's intake phase they contract again and help propel the blood forward. If you touch the skin over an artery you can feel your pulse and can sense the artery's diameter changing rythmically.

► *Measuring Blood Pressure*

In order to measure your blood pressure, the blood flow in the upper arm is stopped by pressure from an inflatable cuff. Then, with a stethoscope, one can hear the blood flow in the bend of the elbow. Gradually, air is let out of the cuff until the highest pressure (known as systolic blood pressure) peaks and pushes past the bottleneck. But the pressure of the cuff is still strong and compresses the artery after every pressure peak, so that the bloodstream can move only in jolts. As the blood vessels open and close, eddies form, which can be heard in the stethoscope as "pulse sounds." If the cuff's pressure is decreased further, a second level is reached where the artery's elasticity can maintain a continual blood flow (the diastolic blood pressure), and the pulsing sound disappears again.

This technique of measuring blood pressure with an inflatable cuff was developed around the turn of the century by Rivarocci, an Italian specialist for internal medicine. Blood pressure is always expressed as a combined value. A measurement of 120/80, for example means a systolic blood pressure of 120 mm of mercury (Hg) and a diastolic blood pressure of 80 mmHg. The pulse tone that is heard through a stethoscope is known as the Korotkov-tone, after its Russian discoverer.

► *What is an Infarction?*

As we age our blood vessels lose elasticity due to arteriosclerosis (the hardening of arteries by calcium deposits). The result is that the pressure peaks increase as our blood vessels grow more rigid. This places considerable stress on the blood vessels and on the heart.

One of the greatest dangers in arteriosclerosis is the complete blockage of a blood vessel. (This is described in detail in chapter 5.) Here we will concentrate on one particular effect of such a blockage: What will happen if the blood stops flowing completely in a certain part of the circulatory system, and if those parts of an organ next to a blockage are no longer supplied with oxygen and nutrients? This is known as an infarction (from the Latin *infarcire:* to block). In everyday language we speak of a "heart attack," or, when the brain is affected a "stroke." Cells that are cut off from the bloodstream in this way will lose their supply of nutrients and soon die.

Whether a blood supply loss with destruction of tissue will remain without consequences or lead to severe disruptions of function including even death, will depend mainly on the extent and importance of the affected region. Blockages in the excitation regions of the heart have particularly dramatic consequences. They can disrupt heart function within minutes or even seconds—the heartbeat deteriorating into irregular spasms (fibrillation) and the blood circulation coming to a stop.

SUMMARY

The words "blood circulation" describe all the blood vessels, including the heart as the central "pumping station." The amount of blood present in the circulatory system is about 9.5 pints (4.5 liters). The pressure in the system is measured using an inflatable cuff and a stethoscope. The pressure varies in the rhythm of the pulse beats between a maximal (systolic) and a minimal (diastolic) value. Arteriosclerosis increases the difference between these extremes, leading to increased stress on the blood vessel walls. A blockage (infarction) can lead to tissue disruptions and—particularly if these involve the heart or brain—can cause death.

►► Our Blood's Composition

Our blood is not a simple liquid like ink or red wine. If blood is placed in a container the difference becomes apparent in a few minutes: The blood which was liquid now changes into a semi-solid mass which can no longer be poured—it has coagulated. After thirty minutes to an hour it becomes obvious that the mass consists of a firm red component and of a yellow liquid part: these are coagulum clot and the blood serum.* A complete separation of the two components is possible only with the help of a centrifuge. At a speed of several thousand revolutions per minute, the clot collects at the bottom of the container, constituting about half of the total volume. The blood serum that floats above is normally clear except after fatty meals, which cause a milky clouding.

Coagulation is a biochemical process. It leads to a clumping together of cells and proteins in our blood and serves to seal breaches in the blood vessels. Certain chemicals, like the salts of citric acid, can be used to prevent the process from taking place in a test tube.

► Blood Serum/Blood Plasma

The term "blood serum" describes only the liquid portion of the blood that remains after the coagulation process is fully completed. By contrast, the uncoagulated blood liquid which normally flows through our body is called plasma. In blood testing it is very important to decide whether the blood is to be left to coagulate, or whether this should be prevented by adding certain chemicals. Some tests can be done only with serum while for others plasma is necessary.

PLASMA COMPONENTS The main component of plasma or serum is water, which makes up about 90 percent. Dissolved in the water are

(*Editor's note: This type of separation is usually done on anticoagulated blood.)

8

proteins (about 8 percent) and salts (about 1 percent). Our blood's main protein is called albumin, and the salt present in the largest amount is sodium chloride (table salt).

The concentration levels of fats and sugars in our blood vary with our diet. In a fasting state the most prevalent fat is cholesterol, at about 0.2 percent of the weight of the blood plasma, and the only significant blood sugar at that time is glucose, at about 0.1 percent.

Proteins, sugars, fats, and salts constitute more than 99.9 percent of all the substances contained in our blood plasma, yet the remaining 0.1 percent include hundreds and even thousands of chemical compounds. And new ones are being discovered every year. These are primarily the signalling substances (hormones and hormone-like substances) which occur in small traces only, as well as a few nutrients (vitamins) which the body cannot synthesize by itself, and finally, waste products of our cell metabolism.

Among these, a metabolic product of our red blood pigment deserves mention: bilirubin, which constitutes only 0.001 percent, but which stands out because of its brilliant yellow color. It is the reason why blood serum is bright yellow. If the concentration of bilirubin in the blood increases, the skin also turns yellow and we speak of jaundice (see p. 118).

▶ Our Blood Corpuscles

Since we have defined blood as an organ and as a part of the body composed of cells, we must be sure to describe the red and white blood cells which manage the blood's two most important functions: transporting oxygen and maintaining "law and order" in the blood.

The number of our blood cells is unimaginably large. Nine and a half pints (4.5 liters) of blood contain around 20 trillion (20,000,000,000,000) red and 20 billion (20,000,000,000) white blood corpuscles. Additionally there are about one trillion platelets which play a part in sealing leaks in our blood vessels. The medical terms are erythrocytes (red blood cells), leukocytes (white blood cells) and thrombocytes (platelets). To speak of blood corpuscles instead of blood cells is quite accurate, especially for erythrocytes and thrombocytes, since they do not possess a nucleus, which is required in defining a body "cell."

LEUKOCYTES Leukocytes do have a nucleus, which allows them to adapt their metabolism to continually changing conditions, and also to reach extreme levels of performance—for example when bacteria enter our body. They are able to achieve this by synthesizing proteins based on genetic information contained in the nucleus. White blood cells come in a variety of subgroups which can be divided into two main types: "feeding cells" (phagocytes) and "guardian cells."

Most important because of their large number among the phagocytes are the granulocytes, which are named after the microscopically small grains (granula) in their interiors which contain a type of digestive juice. They normally constitute 60 to 70 percent of our leukocytes, and have a lifespan of two to three days (unless they die earlier while fighting a defensive battle). Granulocytes literally sacrifice themselves for the organism they are a part of. Once they have gorged themselves with bacteria, soot particles, remains of dead cells, or other substances, they first digest them in their interior and then dissolve themselves. Other important types of feeding cells are monocytes and macrophages.

The second main group of white blood cells are the lymphocytes which we discuss collectively as "guardian cells." Their primary task is to distinguish between substances that are part of our body and those that are foreign. Only about 4 percent of all lymphocytes are found in the bloodflow; most are contained in the lymph nodes immediately adjacent to the blood vessels, as well as in the spleen. Our liver, lungs, and bone marrow also contain these "guardians." There are short-lived lymphocytes with a life expectancy of about one week, as well as long-lived "memory cells" which can live for more than a year.

Lymphocytes perform particularly well in identifying biochemical and structural properties of all the substances and cells which occur in our body, and in memorizing them. Their behavior is analogous to a customs official checking passports: Passengers belonging to the body who are not suspicious are let go, but alien or otherwise "suspicious subjects" (for example cancer cells) are attacked directly or marked with certain proteins (antigens) so that they can be recognized easily by the feeding cells.

▶ *Artificial Blood*

In this age of organ replacements attempts are, of course, also being made to develop "artificial blood." However, the chances for developing a fully lifelike synthetic version of such a complex organ as our blood are small. Until now it has only been possible to create a blood volume replacement, compensating for blood loss by replacing with a liquid. Pure water is unsuitable because it would cause our cells to burst and halt our vital processes. However, if certain salts and proteins or protein substitutes are added to the water it can at least be used to compensate for a small blood loss, or to work long enough to transport someone to a hospital.

Despite intensive research efforts it is still not possible to fully replace human blood with an artificial substance. Apart from mere volume replacement, only real blood with all of its cells, defensive substances, and coagulants can be used to fulfill the organ's many functions.

▶ *Blood Transfusions*

In order to compensate for life-threatening blood losses of more than 30 percent, donor blood is needed. It is usually packaged in pint-sized pouches and stored in "blood banks" from which it can be obtained when needed.

The first transfusion from person to person was attempted in England in 1825. These transfusions often had fatal results which were understood only after the different blood groups and their mutual incompatibility had been discovered around 1900. Today we distinguish four main blood groups, known as A, B, AB and O, which must be matched in transfusions in order to avoid potentially fatal complications. There are also six subgroups of the so-called Rhesus factor system. These are identified by three lower case and three upper case letters (c,d,e,C,D,E). There are also numerous other subgroups identified by such names as "Kell" or "Duffy." Blood properties that are important in the event of a transfusion are recorded in what is known as a "blood passport," which you can get, for example, at a blood donation clinic. Owing to today's safe blood group and compatibility tests, blood transfusions are no longer dangerous. However, problems can arise if the donor suffers from a virus infection (for example AIDS, or certain forms of hepatitis). This means that every blood donation must be carefully examined for the presence of such viruses. For this reason, and in order not to waste the valuable substance blood, great thrift is used in handing out blood. In the U.S.A. blood donations are voluntary and may not be paid for. The cost per unit varies and covers the processing and handling only.

SUMMARY

The blood that circulates in our body is composed of liquid plasma and blood cells. In a test tube blood will coagulate, and the solid portion, the blood clot, settles at the bottom. The remaining uncoagulated liquid is known as serum. Plasma consists of about 90 percent water, 8 percent proteins, and about one percent salts. The remainder are lipids and sugars, hormones, metabolic products, and many other chemical substances. The blood's solid component contains about 20 trillion red blood cells, and 20 billion white blood cells as well as one trillion blood platelets per 9.5 pints (4.5 liters). Red blood cells (erythrocytes) work primarily to transport oxygen, white blood cells serve as defenses, and platelets aid coagulation. A fully functional artificial blood substitute has not yet been developed. When blood is lost it is replaced by a "unit" of donor's blood.

►► *Blood—The Mirror of Biological Equilibrium*

Every single cell of our body is surrounded by a fine web of capillaries. Across its thin walls each cell maintains close contact with the bloodstream. It absorbs different substances from the blood and passes others back into it. These exchange processes cause fluctuations in our blood's composition, which in turn mirror the functional states of our cells and tissues.

A good example are fluctuations in nutrient levels over the course of a day. Their concentration rises after each meal, and, after reaching a peak, decreases to the original value. The increase is caused by the transfer of nutrients from the intestine into the bloodstream, and the decrease is the result of our various body cells using these nutrients. It is theoretically possible to analyze the levels of all nutrients present in a blood sample at any time of day or night, and to give a precise description of our entire organism's absorption and consumption of nutrients.

However, this is not quite as simple to accomplish as it may seem. The level of a substance's concentration that can be measured at any time is determined by two opposing rates of flow: supply rate and absorption rate.

During sports activities, for example, blood sugar is consumed and lactic acid is produced. Our liver supplies fresh sugar while it absorbs and processes excess lactic acid. The concentration in the blood of the two substances, sugar and lactic acid, will depend on the rate of supply and absorption in the muscle and liver. If the effort of the muscle cells exceeds the performance of our liver cells, then our blood sugar level will decrease while the lactic acid concentration will increase. If on the other hand both cell types are working at exactly the same rate, blood values will remain constant, even if both substances are being metabolized in large quantities.

▶ *Fluid Equilibrium (The Steady State)*

The simplest way to demonstrate the steady state principle is to imagine a sink with a partially open drain. If the plug is used to reduce the opening to a few millimeters, and if the faucet is opened half way, the water level will rise very quickly at first, but once it reaches a certain height it remains constant. At this point both supply and drainage rates are exactly even. It is even possible to increase or decrease the supply rate within fairly generous margins without noticeably altering the water level in the basin. This is because of the fluid equilibrium: If the supply rate decreases so does the pressure at the drainage point, if it increases, so does drainage pressure, and with it the amount of fluid drained. Systems with a fluid equilibrium therefore tend to be self-stabilizing at a certain level. Only extreme changes in supply or drainage rates will cause the basin to empty or to overflow.

Our organism possesses many such fluid equilibriums which contribute to keeping the blood's composition, and the various concentration levels of its substances as constant as possible. Similar to the way in which water pressure in a basin influences the drainage rate, our body's metabolic systems adjust their performance levels to changes in supply rate. If, for example, blood sugar concentration is high, the sugar metabolizing rate in the liver increases, and if it is low, it decreases.

Fluid equilibriums are among life's fundamental principles. The law of supply and demand ensures that concentrations of initial substances and of end products do not fluctuate too much—in our blood, in our entire organism, and even in our higher forms of organization, such as the economy.

However, as the comparison with our economy already suggests, the law of supply and demand alone is not enough to maintain an equilibrium in a complex system. Raw materials can be depleted, sudden peaks in demand can catastrophically outstrip supply. When applied to our body's equilibrium and particularly to the maintaining of a constant blood composition this has certain consequences. For example: if food supply fails or if a marathon depletes all our energy reserves, then the fluid equilibrium alone can not maintain a constant blood sugar level, and additional control mechanisms have to come into play.

▶ *Regulatory Mechanisms*

If someone were to close the faucet in our model equilibrium basin, only a water-level sensor could prevent complete drainage, either by closing the drain, or by activating a supplementary reservoir once the water level sinks below a critical level.

The "water-level" sensor of our blood sugar level, for example, is in our pancreas, which controls a powerful regulatory mechanism with the two hormones, insulin and glucagon. Insulin lowers the blood sugar level by increasing our body's sugar consumption, while glucagon elevates blood sugar levels by increasing sugar production from other sources. If during the night our blood sugar falls below a certain level because of a lack of food, the pancreas will register the danger, decrease insulin production, and increase glucagon production. This means that our organism shifts from sugar consumption to sugar production. The blood sugar level increases and a new equilibrium is reached. If in the morning there is a sudden flood of sugar— via the intestine, this too is registered by the pancreas. Hormone production is then shifted from glucagon back to insulin, our body's sugar production is decreased, and the sugar consumption increased.

SUMMARY

The composition of our blood mirrors the state of our entire organism. The measurable concentrations of its various substances are in a state of fluid equilibrium. This means that they are determined by levels of supply and demand, varying only within certain limits that are compatible with our organism's vital needs. If a substance threatens to exceed these limits, certain regulatory mechanisms are activated, including hormones and other messenger substances.

▶▶ *Pathological Variations in Blood Composition*

▶ *The History of Our Blood as a Mirror of Disease*

The idea of using changes in blood composition to draw conclusions about diseases is as old as medicine itself. Even Hippocrates, a Greek physician who lived around 400 B.C., and who is regarded as the father of medicine, suspected that the "bodily fluids," blood and urine were affected by disease. But since he had no knowledge of the blood's components, functions, fluid equilibrium, and regulatory mechanisms, he—like all physicians of the following 2,000 years— had to rely on assumptions. It was not until the end of the 17th century that the chemical and microscopic analysis of our blood were first attempted, and the results connected with certain diseases. Important names in this context are Robert Boyle (1627–1691), Antoin Laurent Lavoisier (1743–1794), Joseph Gay-Lusac (1778–1850), and Jens Jacob von Berzelius (1779–1848). But despite intensive research, Berzelius noted as late as 1840 that no significant difference had been found between the blood of the healthy and the sick. The reason was that the methods available at that time could identify only substance groups, but not individual substances.

Today, 150 years later, we know that it is exceptional for a disease to affect an entire class of substances, such as all of the blood's proteins, and that it was therefore almost impossible to recognize a disease with the coarse chemical and physical methods of that time. There are for example hundreds of different proteins in our blood, and every one requires a special method to determine pathological changes in its level of concentration. Detailed examinations of our blood and its components began in the middle of the last century.

As a rule, a disease will affect certain members of a class of substances, e.g. individual proteins, carbohydrates, hormones, while not affecting other, often very similar substances. Moreover, an initially isolated change in one substance will bring about other, often typical changes in other substances. It is the task of the blood test to find as many typical changes as possible, and to gather the elements from which the physician can construct, as in a mosaic, the complete image of a medical diagnosis.

▶ *The Example of Blood Testing for Diabetes Mellitus*

To give a more detailed introduction to the diagnostic puzzle of blood testing, we will use the example of diabetes mellitus. It will be discussed again in the pages on metabolic disorders.

The majority of measurable changes in the blood of someone suffering from diabetes can be traced back to a single cause: insufficient production or ineffectiveness of insulin, the hormone that lowers blood sugar levels. In a healthy organism, insulin is produced every time the biological sensors of the pancreas detect an increase in blood sugar (glucose) beyond the normal value.

Diabetes causes two typical changes in the blood: Immediately after eating, glucose levels rise more than they would in a non-diabetic person, while insulin levels rise less than normal. The result is that although large amounts of sugar are present, the body's cells cannot metabolize it as long as they have not been stimulated by insulin.

Instead, an excessive amount of fat is metabolized since insulin also regulates our fat metabolism. This leads to other negative effects, including a collecting of fatty acids and their metabolic products known as ketone bodies. Since these acidic substances can be damaging to the cells, the body attempts to flush them out through the kidneys. The result is a loss of both fluid and of salts (electrolytes). In severe cases, this complex disorder can lead to loss of consciousness, coma, and even death.

However, all these biochemical changes do not even begin to describe the diagnostic "mosaic" or puzzle mentioned earlier. Often, insulin production will begin after some delay and will stop the disordered reaction in time by stimulating sugar consumption and by inhibiting fat metabolization. But there are dangers with this process, as well: alarmed by the extremely elevated sugar level (hyperglycemia), the pancreas may react with an excessive production of insulin. As a result, glucose consumption does not stop even during fasting (such as at night) and sugar deficiencies (hypoglycemia) can result. The brain reacts by inducing feelings of ravenous hunger, and the diabetic feels the urge to eat sweets, which starts the vicious cycle all over again.

Blood test results for cases like the one just described can vary widely. They will depend on the phase at which the blood sample was taken and on the severity of the disorder. The blood sugar level may be extremely elevated or extremely depressed, the blood may or may not be highly acidic. A single test value is not sufficient to make any definite statements. Only with a combination of different test results that keep track of changes over the course of an entire day, or by measuring after a test meal can one obtain the "mosaic" pieces that will finally fit into a complete diagnostic picture.

▶ *Mechanisms That Underly Pathological Changes*

Many diseases can be described as deviations from a state of equilibrium. Testing the blood often reveals strong variations between measured values, or an equilibrium which is set at too high or too low levels. These deviations from a balanced state are caused by functional disorders in an entire organ or disruptions of specific organ functions, deficiencies resulting from dietary imbalances, extremely high nutrient consumption rates—caused by a "hungry" tumor, for example, or blood loss. We will discuss the specific disorders of supply and demand balance in detail in relation to each individual disease.

Another fundamental mechanism that causes pathological changes in blood composition is the injection of cell contents from damaged tissue into the bloodstream. With cardiac infarction, for example, the blockage of an artery causes an insufficient supply of blood to the heart muscle, leading to the death of cells in a more or less widespread area. Even if this disruption has no significant impact on heart function and the circulatory system—which would lead to a disturbance in the biological balance—the dying heart muscle cells still empty their cellular contents into the bloodstream. It is by measuring these substances that we can estimate the time and extent of a cardiac infarction.

Both of these mechanisms lead to passive type of disturbances in blood composition, where our blood only mirrors what has occurred in the tissues which surround it like a riverbed. By contrast, the third basic mechanism leading to pathological changes in blood composition is an active reaction by the blood itself to disruptive influences. As we mentioned in the first chapter, blood's functions are mainly tied to its cells, the corpuscles. Erythrocytes transport oxygen, leukocytes provide the means of defense and waste disposal, and thrombocytes repair damage to the circulatory system. Thus our body reacts to increased demands made on one of these systems by increasing the available number of corresponding cell types. These changes in blood composition are not necessarily "pathological," but they signal that our blood cells are reacting to a disturbance in the biological equilibrium.

A well-known example is the increase in blood cells that long-distance athletes experience while training at high altitudes. The oxygen-poor air of mountainous regions stimulates increases in erythrocytes of up to 50 percent in order to permit more storage of oxygen in the blood.

An increased production of leukocytes is usually triggered by a preceding loss, for example, due to a fight against bacteria. As a rule the final result is a measurable increase in cells, but in cases of dramatic cell losses the leukocytes will still be depleted.

A very particular mechanism of cell depletion occurs with the immunodeficiency disease of AIDS. The human immunodeficiency virus (HIV), which triggers the disease, attacks specifically our defensive cells and impedes their reproduction and function (see p. 82).

Over the course of a defensive reaction we may not only find that the total number of a certain cell population has increased or decreased, but also that the defensive substances they produce are accumulating or are depleted as a sign of the struggle. This is true for our antibodies, which are produced by specialized lymphocytes, the so-called plasma cells which serve to mark and destroy foreign organisms and proteins. They frequently remain in the blood for years, indicating whether our organism has come into contact with a certain virus, bacterium, or foreign protein. This can be useful in many ways with blood tests. For example, it can be used to determine the extent to which a population has been contaminated with a certain disease, such as infectious hepatitis, tuberculosis, or AIDS, as well as to test women planning a pregnancy for the necessity of German measles inoculation, or to determine the proteins that trigger allergic hayfever.

SUMMARY

Pathological changes in our body lead to measurable deviations from the normal values for blood composition. Since among the many substances in the blood only a few are affected at a time, blood testing is like a puzzle: the physician determines the levels of many substances and attempts to deduce the underlying disease from the pattern of observable changes. A distinction is made between disruptions of the fluid equilibrium and regulatory mechanisms, the presence of cell contents from destroyed cells, and the reactions of blood cells as part of their defensive actions.

2

FROM BLOOD SAMPLE TO
LABORATORY FINDINGS

Following our—admittedly a little theoretical—introduction to the fundamentals of blood analysis, we will now describe the more practical aspects. The patient's shirt sleeves are rolled up, the physician, nurse, or technician (called a phlebotomist) reaches for the syringe, and what happens next?

▸▸ *Don't Be Afraid of Giving a Blood Sample!*

Does the idea of giving a blood sample make you feel a little queasy, too? Many people faint at the mere sight of blood. Others feel the pain even before the needle has touched their skin. Perhaps it will help you avoid extreme reactions if you know exactly what happens when a blood sample is taken. And if you do belong to those who are prone to fainting from excitement or pain, just ask the technician to let you lie down during the procedure. You will gladly be accommodated.

▸ *The Actual Procedure*

Most commonly, blood samples are taken from the bend of the elbow. Three large and for the most part easily visible veins are situated here immediately beneath the skin: the vena cephalica, vena basilica, and a short connecting blood vessel between the two, the vena mediana cubiti. If you cover your upper arm with your hand and squeeze lightly you should be able to see at least one of them looking like a blue ribbon peering through the skin.

Our veins transport used, oxygen-starved blood back from our body's extremities towards our heart and lungs. In our arm this blood flows upward from our fingertips towards the shoulders. So it can help to cause a slight congestion of the bloodflow just above the elbow by means of a cuff or a piece of rubber hose in order to see the veins more clearly as they become engorged.

The three veins just mentioned carry relatively little blood. The actual main "supply lines" are situated deep inside the arm, and are surrounded by protective layer of muscle and fibrous membranes (muscle fasciae). Here, too, are the arteries that transport oxygen-rich blood from the heart towards our arms and hands. Any danger that a technician might accidentally open a blood vessel large enough for us to bleed significantly is therefore negligible.

The most easily visible veins are not always the ones best suited to taking a blood sample. The phlebotomist will prefer a thick, easily palpable vein even if it is invisible under the skin.

Once a suitable place to take the sample has been found it is cleaned with a disinfecting agent, usually alcohol. Unless, of course, the sample is intended to determine your blood alcohol level, in which case a different agent is used.

At last the time has come: The technician places a sterile needle on the syringe, pierces the skin by using gentle but firm pressure and pushes the tip of the needle about half an inch (a centimeter) into the vein. It is not due to malice that the needle is not the thinnest type available, but rather the slightly thicker standard diameter. If the needle were too thin, its sharp tip might pierce the other wall of the blood vessel more easily, and the result would be a futile pricking as well as a bruise.

Strangely, sometimes the prick can hardly be felt and sometimes it is extremely painful. Whether the prick feels painful or not depends on whether one of the skin's tactile organs has been touched by the needle. Unfortunately, these pain receptors are microscopically small and completely invisible. The chances for slipping between them at the elbow and forearm are fairly good, but at the back of the hands they are placed so densely that one of them will almost always be hit.

WHAT IF NO BLOOD FLOWS? Once the needle tip is placed properly inside the vein, blood can be removed with a Vacutainer® (vacuum cartridge) which creates the necessary suction. Sometimes despite a perfectly placed needle no blood or very little blood flows.

There are various possible reasons. Very thin veins are easily sucked against the needle's opening by the pressure differential and in this way seal the tip. Occasionally the needle comes to rest at a vein valve, which will prevent the blood's flowing away from the heart. Finally, the needle may encounter a blood clot that might have been left behind at the site of a previous blood sample. In all of these cases the technician will try to get the blood flowing again by gently moving the needle forward or backward, or sometimes by lessening the amount of suction. Once the needle is withdrawn from the vein, its wall will close itself within a minute or two with the clotting mechanism we have already mentioned. To prevent residual bleeding during that time the technician usually presses a gauze pad firmly against the tiny hole.

▶ *Taking Blood Samples for Different Tests*

If a variety of blood tests will be done, the technician usually removes the Vacutainer® from the syringe and needle which remain in the vein, and replaces it with another in order to obtain more blood. The reason is not necessarily that the lab needs these large quantities. It is more likely that the different tubes will contain different additives. As we have mentioned, some tests are conducted using coagulated blood while others use uncoagulated blood. In order to inhibit the natural clotting process, specially prepared vacuum tubes are used which contain, for example, certain salts of citric acid as an anticoagulant.

Exchanging syringes while the needle stays in place used to be an awkward and fairly "bloody" affair. Today most technicians use special blood sampling systems that fill automatically once they are attached to the needle valve, and do not need the technician's intervention.

Important note: All of this costs money, of course. Systems that use needle valves and vacuum cartridges cost more than conventional one-way plastic syringes, and these in turn cost more (and cause more waste) than the traditional glass syringes and steel needles which were cleaned and sterilized after each blood sample.

However, when taking blood samples price alone cannot determine which system should be used. With reused syringes there is a certain risk of infection, because blood is the carrier for dangerous diseases—particularly hepatitis and the immunodeficiency disease AIDS.

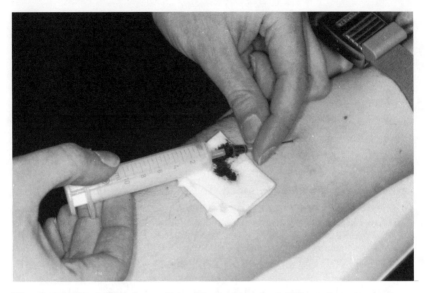

Blood sampling using the traditional, open method. When changing syringes with the needle in place a few drops of blood are always lost.

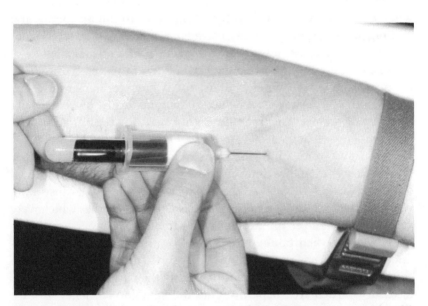

Blood sampling using a closed vacuum method. The vacuum cartridge fills automatically. No blood is lost when syringes are changed.

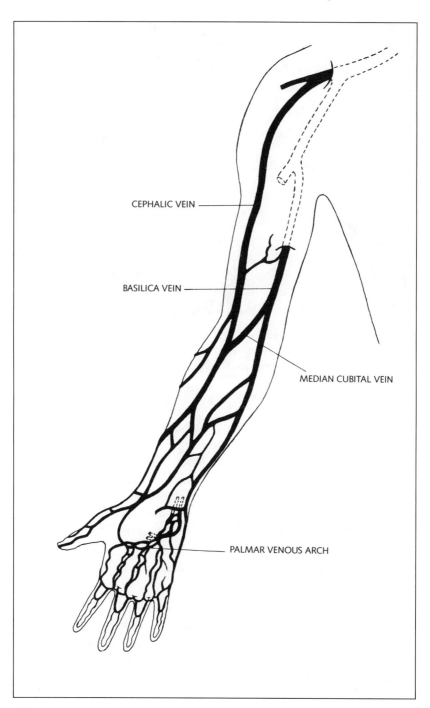

CEPHALIC VEIN

BASILICA VEIN

MEDIAN CUBITAL VEIN

PALMAR VENOUS ARCH

The most important surface veins of the upper arm

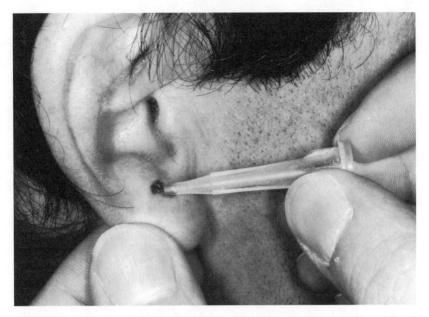

Samples taken from the earlobe or the fingertips contain capillary blood. These are used primarily to determine blood sugar levels. (Editor's note: In babies, blood is often drawn from the heel.)

▶ *Blood Samples from Fingertips or Earlobes*

It is not always necessary to take blood from a vein for a blood analysis. For example, to determine blood sugar levels capillary blood, the blood from our smallest, hair-like blood vessels can be used. These blood vessels can be seen only under a magnifying glass and cannot easily be punctured individually. It is sufficient to pierce a well-irrigated section of skin on the earlobes or fingertips with a sharp lancet, and to collect the resulting drop of blood with a fine glass tube.

SUMMARY

Blood samples for laboratory testing are usually taken from a surface vein of the elbow with a vacuum cartridge. For some tests, such as blood sugar level analysis, a drop of capillary blood from finger tips or earlobes can be used. For certain tests blood is prevented from clotting by using chemical additives.

►► *What Happens to the Blood in the Laboratory?*

Once our blood sample has been taken it is prepared for analysis. It is rare for a blood sample to be usable for testing as is. As a rule, it is left to coagulate fully until the liquid serum and the solid blood clot containing the cells have separated. This takes ten to twenty minutes. However, if a patient has been treated with anticoagulants, this process can take a lot longer—much to the lab's displeasure, since blood clotting over a period of several hours may obstruct needles and wires of the expensive analysis machinery.

► *Separating Serum and Blood Clot (Coagulum)*

As we have mentioned above, in order to obtain pure serum it is not enough to let the blood sit until the coagulum has completely settled. A centrifuge has to be used, and a fairly high number of revolutions is needed for the liquid and solid blood components to separate completely.

Under standard conditions the centrifugal force causes a one thousand to three thousand-fold increase in the blood clot's weight, pushing it to the bottom within ten minutes. How can a centrifuge withstand these strong forces? Simply by virtue of always being loaded with two roughly equal-sized containers. This way their weights balance each other and the rotor axis is not overstressed.

After centrifuging the serum is used for further analysis. If the blood has been treated with anticoagulants the remaining fluid is called plasma. Unlike serum it still contains clotting proteins and is therefore well suited to testing coagulation processes. The blood clot (coagulum) is usually not used because centrifuging damages the blood cells. The concentrate can only be used to determine blood groups. Most other blood cell analyses—collectively known as "blood picture" (or blood count)—are made using uncentrifuged, anticoagulated blood.

► *Blood Sedimentation*

Finally there is one other special test, called "blood sedimentation," in which blood cells and plasma are separated without the help of a centrifuge. Here the blood which has been prevented from coagulating by a special additive is placed in a thin glass tube and left standing in an upright position. The time is then measured in which the solid

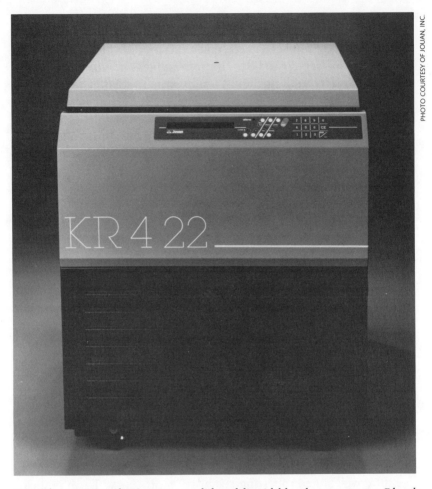

Centrifuges are used to separate solid and liquid blood components. Blood cells are pushed to the bottom by a force equal to 1,000–3,000 times their own weight.

blood components sink to the bottom. This method was standardized at the beginning of this century by the Swedish internist Alf Westergren. The normal sedimentation rate according to Westergren is about 5 to 10 millimeters an hour and is somewhat higher in women than in men.

To this day it is not known exactly how pathological processes affect sedimentation rate, but it has been known for a long time that some diseases lead to an increase and others to a decrease in sedimentation rate. Very high sedimentation rates often point to an infection—a battle between our organism and substances from within the body, from the outside, or against dead or transformed cells.

SUMMARY

To prepare for most tests, blood is centrifuged in the lab to separate the serum or plasma from the blood cells. In blood sedimentation the rate at which blood cells settle spontaneously is used to detect infectious processes.

▶ *Final Preparations*

Frequently the technician taking the blood sample does not conduct the actual tests but involves a specialist instead. This means that the sample must be packed so that it cannot break and be damaged. Many blood components change relatively quickly once they are removed from the biological cycle and are exposed to air, light, or heat. The physician has to know precisely what conditions must be maintained for each specific test. If the lab is situated far away, samples may have to be sent refrigerated, or even in special cases packed in carbon dioxide ice (dry ice) at −108°F (−78°C).

All the preparatory work we have described so far, from taking the blood sample to its arrival in the lab is collectively known as preanalytics (from the Latin *prae:* before). Next comes the actual blood analysis which results in a measurement.

▶▶ *Old and New Measuring Methods*

"Measuring and weighing": these two terms have always been at the core of scientific work. The more medical practitioners have developed away from being "medicine men" into the scientifically patterned physicians of our time, the more have exact methods of measurement come to be at the center of their work. No field of medical specialization demonstrates this more clearly than laboratory medicine.

Today classic measuring devices like rulers and scales are of little use since the objects to be measured are at most a few micrometers in diameter. (A micrometer is one thousandth of a millimeter, or 0.0000394 inches.) Blood cells and some bacilli can be seen and classified under a microscope. All other blood components, such as proteins and fat molecules, are only millionths of millimeters in size and cannot be seen under a microscope. Instead, we are dealing with the "submicroscopic" size range.

▶ The Light Microscope

The microscope was invented as long as 400 years ago by a Dutchman named Jansen. It consists of a system of optical lenses which permit an object to be magnified from 100 to 1,000 times its original size. A blood platelet (thrombocyte) or a bacterium with a diameter of a micrometer (one thousandth of a millimeter) appears one millimeter in size when magnified 1,000 times—enough to be seen clearly.

The much finer interior structures of these cells can only be examined with an electron microscope, a much more sophisticated device that is rarely used in daily practice.

▶ Blood Cell Analysis

The microscopic analysis of blood cells has been known for 200 years. In order to examine them, a few drops of blood are mixed with a diluting agent and possibly a dye, placed inside a tiny glass chamber (counting chamber), and magnified under a microscope. Apart from their number the physician is also interested in the type of cells present and any variations in the cells' size or shape. For this, a drop of blood is spread on a glass slide, dried, and stained. The stain will cause the cell nucleus to appear purple, and the surrounding cell body a reddish color.

The determination of blood cells according to number, size, and shape is known as "blood count." A chemical analysis of blood liquids is not part of this. A complete blood count includes cell counts, red blood pigment (hemoglobin), and red blood cell volume (hematocrit), as well as an analysis of all cells according to type, shape, size and affinity for stains. The daily workload makes extreme demands on the ability of staff to perform these manually. For this reason more and more modern techniques are being developed to examine cells and their detailed structures with the help of automation.

THE USE OF AUTOMATION AND COMPUTERS One widely used technique for automated blood particle analysis can be found in what are known as "blood count machines." A blood sample is sucked into a glass tube through a tiny opening across which runs an electric field. Every time a blood cell passes the opening—which at normal rates of flow happens hundreds and thousands of times every second—it causes a change in the electric field that is registered by the machine. The number of electrical impulses that are measured is equivalent to the number of blood cells contained in the blood sample, while the amount of voltage indicates the cells' size. An extremely fast computer program is used to compute from the different numbers and intensities of impulses how many cells of what size were contained in the blood sample.

Apart from electrical impulses, refracted light, as well as fluorescence and other physical principles of measurement, can be used to record the number, size, and structure of individual cells. These modern techniques permit insights into the structures and properties of cells that go far beyond what the human eye can recognize with a microscope.

The analysis of cells—whether by eye and a microscope or by sophisticated machines—is only a small section of the whole field of blood analysis. By far the greatest number of processes which are studied take place submicroscopically, in a dimension that cannot be made visible even with the most sensitive microscopes. Neither the entering of liver enzymes into the bloodstream, nor the strong variations in blood sugar levels of a diabetic can in any way be visibly recorded—the only useful methods are those of chemistry and biochemistry.

SUMMARY

The examination of blood cells, known as a blood count or blood picture, is conducted in the laboratory with the help of a light microscope which shows details at 100- to 1,000-fold magnification. For this a drop of blood is either placed inside a tiny glass chamber or spread on a glass slide and stained. Cells are examined for number, size, shape, and affinity for stains. More recently, electronic methods are being used increasingly in order to make blood pictures simpler and safer to obtain.

▶ *Chemistry: The Science of Molecules*

Chemistry is the science of the tiny components of animate and inanimate nature known as atoms and molecules. For those whose chemistry lessons are a distant memory: a molecule is what we call an aggregation of similar or dissimilar atoms. A compound of two hydrogen atoms with the symbol H, and one oxygen atom with the symbol O, for example, is known as water (H_2O). A compound of twelve hydrogen atoms, six oxygen atoms, and six carbon atoms is called glucose ($C_6H_{12}O_6$). Molecules can be made up of hundreds or even thousands of atoms but they always remain submicroscopically small. Only when millions or billions of similar molecules combine do they become visible.

An important task of clinical chemistry is to develop methods by which extremely small amounts of molecules can be detected. In analyzing blood the detection of a substance in minute amounts is essential, because many vitally important substances are present in our entire blood supply in the thousandth or millionth part of a gram.

Between one or two centuries ago the only reliable device for measuring weight was the scale. The substance to be studied was first isolated from the many surrounding chemical compounds and then measured. Obviously an analysis of chemical blood components was impossible with such coarse methods.

During the last century it was discovered that some blood molecules combine with other molecules in a test tube and display certain characteristic color changes. Bilirubin, for example, which is responsible for jaundice, forms a purple dye when sulfanilic acid is added, and creatinine, which increases in patients with kidney disease, turns bright yellow when combined with picric acid.

The discovery of chemical dye-reactions has enabled us to recognize invisibly tiny molecules with the naked eye, if only indirectly by the dye they have produced. It was easy to demonstrate that the amount of the substance being investigated and the intensity of the resulting dye were directly related: the more of a substance was present, the more intense would be the color. Such color comparisons permitted estimating the approximate amount of a substance. Until the middle of this century color comparisons were a common diagnostic method.

The problems raised by these rule-of-thumb measurements are obvious: measured results depend strongly on the color sense of the

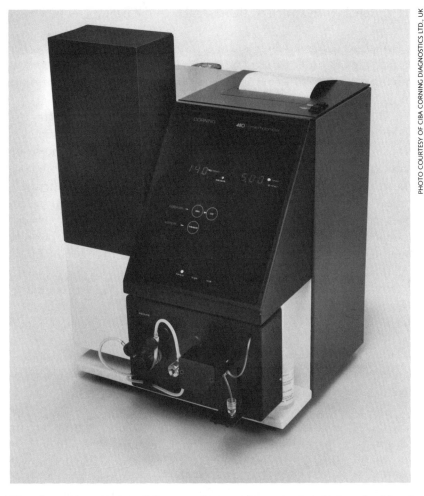

PHOTO COURTESY OF CIBA CORNING DIAGNOSTICS LTD., UK

The photometer is one of the most important measuring devices for blood testing. Blood and color reagent are placed in a cuvette. The resulting color is measured by a photocell.

examiner, tint and intensity of light in the lab, and many other factors. It would be all too easy to obtain a different value in the bright midday sun and during a reddish sunset. Attempts at measuring colors objectively were aided by an important invention made during the 19th century: the photometer.

HOW A PHOTOMETER WORKS   A modern photometer consists essentially of a light source, a glass container, called the cuvette, for the stained liquid that is to be tested, and a photocell which emits an electrical signal when struck by light, similar to the light meter in a camera.

Also needed is a whole series of filters, lenses, prisms, and other optical aids in order to regulate the light used for measuring, and to point it as sharply focussed as possible across the cuvette and onto the photocell.

The more intensely the content of the cuvette is stained, the less light of a certain color will it permit to pass, and the less signal is transmitted by the photocell. We can easily imitate the process by shining a light through a glass filled with diluted ink: the more concentrated the ink is, the less we can see of the light source. The theoretical connections between intensity of light and pigmentation had been discovered as early as the 18th century by the Swiss physicist Lambert, and the German opthalmologist Beer, but it took another hundred years before Lambert-Beer's Law became a part of blood analysis.

OTHER WAYS TO OBTAIN EXACT MEASUREMENTS For completeness' sake we should mention that although staining and light measuring constitute a central measuring principle in chemical blood analysis, there are many other physical and chemical means that can be used to obtain exact measurements. For example, potentiometry which records ions, and radioactivity measurement, is a highly sensitive method to detect hormones or vitamins.

We should also remember that in earlier times not only the eye but also our sense of smell was used as a diagnostic tool. The fruity aroma on a diabetes patient's breath, for example, foretold an imminent loss of consciousness. In this case our nose proved a very fine instrument for detecting acetone bodies—chemical substances which are formed when blood sugar is only partially metabolized. Today the examiner's sensory organs play an ever smaller role due to the progressive automatization of blood chemistry analysis.

Recently some measuring methods have made their mark in blood analysis by making use of the extreme sensitivity of certain biological systems. They involve combining chemical dyes with protein molecules, particularly enzymes and antibodies. These help our organism to detect and process different biological substances—an ability which they retain even in a test tube. The use of such molecules in blood testing has created completely new areas of specialization within laboratory diagnostics. They are called clinical enzymology and immunochemistry.

In 1956 Berson and Yalow were recognized for finding ways of using these remarkable properties of our immune system in examining biological substances. The method they developed to detect the hormone insulin involved antigens that had been marked by radioactivity. Apart from what today are known as radio-immune assays, (or RIA), there are a number of immunochemical measuring methods which require no radioactivity and are known by acronyms such as ELISA.

SUMMARY

Our blood liquids, plasma, or serum, are examined mainly by chemical or biochemical methods. One common principle of measuring involves mixing the blood sample with chemicals which change color on contact with certain blood components. The color is measured with a "photometer," a device that measures light electronically. These days the chemicals used in color measuring are increasingly combined with biological substances, in particular enzymes and antibodies, in order to make a more sensitive analysis.

▶▶ *Blood Testing with Automation*

While in the classic medical disciplines—for example, in surgery or internal medicine—the physician's dexterity and powers of observation are still very important, since the 1960's laboratory diagnostics has developed into an increasingly mechanized discipline. Automatic devices and computers dominate, particularly in large laboratories doing more than ten thousand blood tests every day, because these machines can conduct most tests more quickly and accurately than human operators.

Unlike manual tests for example, modern automated machines require only a few microliters of blood for an analysis. That amount is too small to accurately measure by eye. The accuracy of dosimeters allows the contents of a single, small syringe to be used for multiple tests. Their organizational performance in "stacking" different tests is also remarkable. Controlled by a computer they are able to use every free moment during one chemical reaction to prepare other tests.

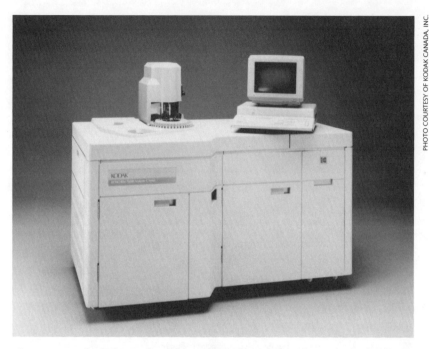

PHOTO COURTESY OF KODAK CANADA, INC.

Computerized machines dominate today's large labs. They can do in minutes what would take human operators hours to accomplish.

▶ Birth of the Autoanalyzer

The first laboratory machine, which was introduced in 1954, and known as a single-channel device, could only perform one test (for example blood sugar level analysis), on a number of different blood samples. Although it has been out of use for years its manufacturer's name, Autoanalyzer, has become the term used for all subsequent analysis machines, just as Xerox and Scotch tape have become generic terms. The first autoanalyzer was able to independently measure out blood, mix blood and reagents, monitor reaction times, conduct photometric measurements, and convert measured signals into laboratory values. The remarkable fact is that it did all this without the help of a computer.

By placing a number of single-channel devices in sequence the first of the multi-channel devices were created, and these dominated clinical chemistry during the 1970's. They were non-selective, which means that they conducted every test that they were capable of on every blood sample. With a total of more than 30 channels these laboratory "dinosaurs" began to produce more superfluous data than necessary measurements. This did not help make lab diagnostics more economical and created a controversy among physicians, medical insurance companies and politicians.

Finally, during the 1980's what we know as the selective analyzers were developed, and these selected only those measurement channels that were actually needed. A prerequisite for the development of this "machine intelligence" was the rapid development of microelectronics. Modern machines now instantly conduct every required test on every sample in a process that is controlled and monitored to the smallest detail. This requires a minimum of time while achieving a maximum of accuracy. For patients and physicians this means a significant improvement in diagnostic possibilities. Particularly in hospitals, but even for general practitioners who are affiliated with a lab, determining blood values involves hardly more effort than measuring blood pressure. As a result, blood tests have become as commonplace in medical practice as listening to the heart and looking into the patient's mouth.

▸▸ *Self-Monitoring—A New Trend*

Perhaps as a reaction to the large machines, a new trend in blood testing has appeared since the 1980's which may soon benefit more patients directly. This is the use of compact, handheld measuring devices that are extremely easy to use due to their sophisticated electronics, permitting blood analysis at any time, anywhere.

The catchphrase for this new technology is "dry chemistry." It enables even physicians with no lab of their own to conduct sophisticated blood tests. For certain tests, such as blood sugar level analysis, it even means that patients can measure their own blood values.

▸ *What is "Dry Chemistry"?*

This method uses a plastic strip or plate on which the required chemicals have been placed in a dry state and sealed—hence the name "dry chemistry." The actual chemical reaction, however, takes place in a liquid solution just as in conventional blood analysis, known as liquid chemistry. The difference is that the necessary liquid is not added by a complicated dosimeter but is supplied by the blood itself.

In urine-testing this technique has existed for years in the form of

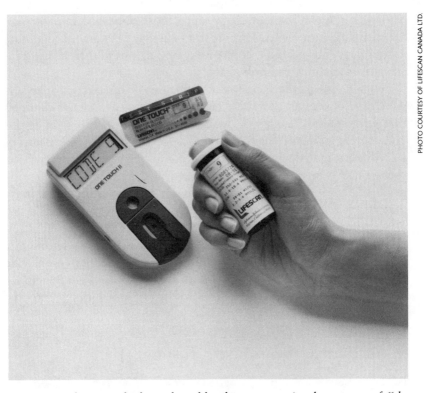

Automatic devices which analyze blood on test strips by means of "dry chemistry" are especially useful in measuring blood sugar levels. They are widely used by patients monitoring their own blood values.

the well-known urine test strip. These strips contain a number of small fields which change color in various ways when they come into contact with urine. The fields' color intensity is then compared to a color scale printed on the package, which allows you to determine with the naked eye whether the urine contains sugar or protein.

Simple yes/no decisions like "protein present" or "protein not present" can be made without electronic measuring devices. But simple color scale comparisons cannot determine exactly how many milligrams of protein are present in a blood or urine sample. Besides, the amount of blood is much too small for a test strip to be immersed in.

TEST STRIP CONSTRUCTION Dry chemical test strips are constructed so as to allow the exact analysis of one single drop of blood inside a measuring device. The test fields consists of different layers, each of which is intended for a particular purpose. The topmost, net-like layer, for example, will retain blood cells if these have not already been removed by centrifuging.

A second spongy layer is designed to absorb a precise amount of plasma, usually a few millionths of a liter in which the sealed chemicals dissolve and react with the substance to be measured. Depending on the method, other layers may be added, for example, to filter out intervening substances.

Dry chemical reactions, just as in liquid chemistry, lead to the formation of a dye whose intensity is proportional to the amount of the substance in question. It is much more difficult than in liquid chemistry to measure the exact intensity of the color since light cannot penetrate the many layers of the test strip. To measure the light reflected by the test area's surface requires sophisticated electronics.

As complicated as all this may sound, using such a dry chemical device is in fact very simple. To determine blood sugar levels you obtain a drop of blood by lightly pricking a fingertip, and then you use a fine tube to place the blood on the test area of a sugar test strip and start the measuring device by pushing a button. The unit then displays cues as when to feed the test strip into the measuring slot, and when to read the results.

Since regular blood sugar level monitoring can be of vital importance for diabetics, special blood sugar measuring devices have been developed quickly and are now widely available. In most cases the cost is covered by the medical insurance. Tests for cholesterol and liver enzymes have also been developed. Cholesterol tests are frequently offered by dispensaries and mobile test units. It should be pointed out, however, that they are not as safe and accurate as conventional liquid chemistry, and that individual tests are relatively expensive due to their technical complexity.

SUMMARY

While blood tests were once conducted manually they now involve more and more computer-controlled machines that are extremely fast and accurate, and require only a few microliters (millionths of liters) of blood for each analysis. The first such machine was the Autoanalyzer which was introduced in 1956. Towards the late 1980's miniaturized test strip analyzing devices appeared on the market. This technology is known as "dry chemistry" and is generally suitable for patients who want to monitor their own blood values.

3

FROM BLOOD COUNT TO
DIAGNOSIS

A blood count is not a finding, and a finding does not constitute a diagnosis. It is a long way from a basic measurement, like
the one provided by an automatic analyzer, to the correct diagnosis of
a disease, and it requires a great deal of specialized medical knowledge. Of course, we cannot attempt to impart all that knowledge
here. But we can explain enough of the foundations of laboratory diagnostics for you to understand why a certain blood count was done.
You will also learn to understand the connections between the numbers in the laboratory test result and your physician's diagnosis. And
you will be able to recognize the difference between normal blood
count values and those indicating a sickness. First, we must explain
the difference between the three terms "measured value," "finding,"
and "diagnosis."

▶ *Measured Value*

A measured value is a technical unit of measurement, a number
without any direct medical reference, for example, "blood sugar 200
mg/dl" (milligrams per deciliter, with a deciliter being one tenth of a
liter). For the physician this can mean a significant though not life-
threatening increase in blood sugar level. To us, measures such as
pounds and ounces are more familiar than the clinical chemical units
"mol," "millimol," "micromol," and so on. The mol takes into ac-

count the number and weight of atoms in a compound, for example, that a molecule of blood sugar is composed of six carbon and oxygen atoms as well as twelve hydrogen atoms.

▶ The Laboratory Findings

How does the technical unit known as a measured value become medically significant? We will use alcohol as an example. We know that a blood alcohol level of 0.9 grams per liter will usually severely affect one's ability to concentrate and to drive safely. But chronic alcoholics can still walk, even at levels of 3 and 4 grams per liter, while someone who rarely consumes alcohol would be suffering from massive poisoning. Thus, the measured value of 0.9 becomes a finding when it is understood in the medical context of the whole person.

The example a blood sugar level of 200 mg/dl (or 10 mmol/l) becomes medically significant as a result of the fact that a healthy person exhibits values around 100 mg/dl (5 mmol/l), and that the dreaded diabetic coma—a particular form of deep loss of consciousness—rarely appears at values of less than 400 mg/dl (20 mmol/l). Here the finding would be that the "blood sugar level is significantly increased but not acutely life-threatening."

▶ The Medical Diagnosis

Various findings eventually contribute to a "diagnosis." We define as findings any objectively measurable signs that could be connected with a disease. They include not only lab findings but also other indicators, such as an increase in blood pressure, an enlarged or hardened liver, and abnormal EKG wave (electrocardiogram) readings. Giving a diagnosis means correctly identifying and naming a disease. A diagnosis can almost never be made on the basis of lab findings alone. It requires a great deal of specialized knowledge and medical experience.

SUMMARY

Identifying a disease with the help of a blood test involves three steps. First, a measured value is obtained. This is a purely technical value and consists of a number and a unit of measurement (e.g. grams/liter). This measured value is examined with all related medical aspects and then becomes a finding. The determining factor is a comparison to measured values in healthy and sick persons. A number of findings finally lead to a diagnosis of the disease, to which other findings such as blood pressure and EKG also contribute.

▶▶ Normal and Ideal Ranges

The example of blood sugar shows how important it is to be aware of healthy blood sugar levels. Only with this knowledge can a finding be derived from a measured value: a measured value of 100 mg/dl is completely normal, a value of 200 mg/dl on the other hand is considered to be pathologically elevated. Where then is the boundary? Is 150 mg/dl still normal, or does it indicate a case of diabetes?

▶ The Normal Range

In order to determine these boundaries a normal range has to be established for every substance that is measured in our blood. To this end the values of several hundred healthy persons are measured and the frequency with which they appear is recorded. The simplest method is to keep a check-list. For example, if we find that after breakfast most healthy persons have blood sugar levels of 100 mg/dl, we see that almost as many have values of 99 mg/dl and 101 mg/dl, while slightly fewer have 98 mg/dl and 102 mg/dl. In this way the frequency decreases for higher and lower values until only a few values of less than 80 mg/dl or more than 120 mg/dl are found. This is shown in the distribution curve in the diagram. This law was discovered 150 years ago by Friedrich Gauss, the German mathematician, and it is true for all such distribution curves. This is why they are referred to as Gaussian standard distribution curves. They are among the most important laws of statistics. They allow predictions for random event series, and are also used in determining normal ranges for blood values.

Mathematically inclined readers may be interested to know that the curve enclosing the distributed values can be computed by using "Gauss's standard deviation formula." In connection with blood tests, Gauss's theory states that the further an individual's blood value deviates from the most common, or middle value, the less likely

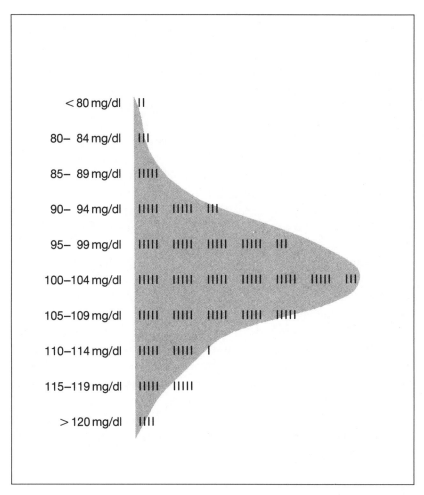

Distribution of blood sugar levels in a group of healthy persons

it is to belong to a healthy person. That possibility cannot be entirely excluded even if values deviate extremely, but with Gauss's curve we can compute when the probability reaches 90, 95, or 99 percent, and when the value cannot be considered healthy any more.

► *The Normal Range Includes Only 95% of Healthy People*

In medicine we include in the "normal range" the values obtained from 95 percent of all healthy persons, even if the distribution of values does not completely correspond to a Gaussian standard distribution curve. The agreement to use 95 percent as the measure of probability is the result of a necessary compromise between the desire to distinguish as clearly as possible between normal and disease values on the one hand, and the need to avoid overly large boundary regions in which "disease" is more probable than "health" on the other hand.

As with any compromise, there are disadvantages. If one considers every value that falls outside of this normal range as a sign of disease, one runs the risk of diagnosing a disease in five percent of the population. And this, after all, would mean every twentieth person who is probably completely healthy. This demonstrates how much physicians, and even more lay persons, whose medical knowledge is limited in scope, have to guard against placing too much importance on, or worse, basing a diagnosis on a single measured value. So we repeat yet again that a diagnosis and the identification of a disease, can be derived only from a combined examination of findings and a patient's history, and never from a single measurement. A blood value which falls outside the normal range is only one stone in the mosaic of a sickness. An isolated value that is slightly increased or decreased may have no meaning at all.

The more a measurement falls outside the limits of the normal range, however, the more attention should be paid to it. In describing individual sicknesses in the next chapters we hardly ever give definite numerical values. Instead we usually mention percentages of deviation or "multiples of normal range values." These statements will refer to the upper or lower limits of a range. If the normal blood sugar value falls in a range between 70 and 100 mg/dl, an increase to "five times normal value" means a value of 500 mg/dl.

► *Ideal Ranges*

In some cases the terms "health" or "normality" are difficult to define, particularly if a blood measurement suggests an imminent disease that has not yet manifested itself. The normal range of values for the blood lipid cholesterol for example is up to 220 mg/dl, meaning that 95 percent of all healthy people have blood values up to this limit. We know on the other hand that "healthy" people with a cholesterol count of 220 mg/dl are more likely in later life to suffer from a heart attack than those with values of, for example, 150 mg/dl. In such special cases it would be better not to define a normal range but rather to indicate an "ideal range," where the values should remain in order to minimize the future risk of a disease. For cholesterol this ideal range reaches up to 200 mg/dl. (It must be recognized that in other population groups, for example, Chinese living in China, the normal values are considerably lower and that such groups are known to have less atherosclerosis.)

▶▶ *Our Metabolism and its Products*

▶ *Nutrients and Their Waste (Catabolic) Products*

As early as a hundred years ago, among the substances measured in our blood and in our other bodily fluids nutrients and their catabolic (from the Greek *kata:* apart) products were the most common. The sum total of our body's chemical transformations, from the resorption of substances by eating and breathing, to digestion, oxydization, storage, and ending with excretion, is called metabolism. And diseases based on a disorder in the regulation of these processes are called metabolic diseases. Given the large number of metabolic processes it is no surprise that measuring their initial substances as well as their intermediate and end products plays an important part in blood testing even today.

These many substances are divided according to their chemical or biological properties into the following five categories: carbohydrates, lipids (fats), proteins, minerals, and gases.

Carbohydrates are sugar and related substances.

Lipids include mainly cholesterol and "neutral fats," as well as their derivatives.

Proteins, as well as serum globulins, are albumin.

Minerals are the different blood salts—primarily sodium chloride, i.e., table salt.

Lastly there are the gases, oxygen and carbon dioxide, which are bound in our blood.

Below we will give a general description of the substances used for measurement. A more detailed discussion of their diagnostic significance is included in the descriptions of individual illnesses.

▶ *Carbohydrates*

Among the carbohydrates in our blood, blood sugar (glucose) is the most important subject of measurement. It is more important for diagnosing diseases of the carbohydrate metabolism than all other sugars and metabolic sugar products combined. Blood sugar measurement is also the most frequently done medical lab test, and is used to detect the most common metabolic disorder, diabetes mellitus.

The chemical formula for glucose is $C_6H_{12}O_6$. This explains the term carbohydrate, which loosely means "carbon water" (from the Greek *hydor:* water). All carbohydrates contain as many carbon atoms (the chemical symbol C) as they do water molecules (the chemical symbol H_2O). Their structural formulas are therefore expressed with such symbols as $C_6H_{12}O_6$ or $C_5H_{10}O_5$.

Compared to glucose, all the other sugar types, such as fruit sugar (fructose) or milk sugar, (lactose) have little significance in standard blood testing. For diagnostic purposes, a certain metabolic product of glucose is far more important. This is the salt of lactic acid, known chemically as lactate (from the Latin *lac:* milk). It is present in the blood at elevated levels not only in severe cases of diabetes and in states of shock but also after physical exertion. An excess of lactate can lead to a dangerous overacidification of our blood.

▶ *Lipids*

Lipids, generally speaking, are substances that do not easily dissolve in water. In chemical terms, they contain fewer oxygen atoms (with the chemical symbol O) than the more easily soluble carbohydrates. The best-known lipid, cholesterol, has the structural formula, $C_{17}H_{16}O$, which means that beside 17 carbon atoms and 16 hydrogen atoms it contains only a single oxygen atom.

Lipids are important particularly for detecting early abnormalities which lead to arteriosclerosis and heart attacks. The most important tests are the cholesterol measurements which are conducted millions of times, throughout the world, as part of public health campaigns in an effort to prevent heart attacks and other arteriosclerotic disorders. Neutral fats, known as triglycerides, are measured almost as often, although their significance for heart attacks is not quite as great. For both cholesterol and triglycerides a measured value of less than 200 mg/dl is considered medically acceptable. If values are higher, further tests are necessary to determine the risk of a possible heart attack.

Lipids provide a particularly good example to show the difference between a value, a finding, and a diagnosis. A cholesterol level of 250 mg/dl, taken by itself has no diagnostic significance. Only in connection with further blood test results, blood pressure measurements, and information from the patient about habits such as smoking, family history, and forms of exercise, can one determine whether this value must be considered excessively high.

The connections between blood lipids and arteriosclerosis are complex, and in many details they baffle even specialists. It is no surprise, therefore, that medical publications—and even more the popular press—publish opposing and confusing statements about the significance of lipid measurements. In order to clarify these contradictory statements it is important to make a distinction between the two different forms in which lipids appear in our blood. They are known by their acronyms HDL (high density lipoproteins) and LDL (low density lipoproteins).

Important in determining the risk of cardiac infarction is not the total cholesterol level in the blood, but rather the cholesterol present in the low density lipoproteins, LDL. The HDL share is in fact regarded as risk-reducing. Many publications refer only to a "total cholesterol level," which may explain some of the apparent contradictions in the literature. Other lipoproteins that are important for cardiac infarction risk levels are known as IDL (intermediate density lipoproteins) and Lp(a).

The different forms in which lipids appear are connected to their low solubility in water. They have to be wrapped between more easily soluble molecules, particularly proteins, to prevent them from swimming in the blood like fat globules in a bowl of soup. Depending on the relative proportion of lipids and proteins, the density of these compound molecules known as "lipoproteins" is higher or lower. This explains such terms as HDL (high density) and LDL (low density).

▶ *Proteins*

Proteins are the most common class of substances in our blood. Their multiplicity is the result of their chemical composition. Much as the way in which words are made with letters, proteins are made up of a number of amino acids.

Human proteins contain 20 different amino acids, which means that their number is roughly comparable to the number of letters in the Latin alphabet. Thus, the number of possible protein combinations approximates the number of words contained in a language written in this alphabet. In fact, biochemistry has already detected thousands of different proteins with widely different amino acid sequences.

This of course leads to interesting questions: How can our body distinguish all of these different proteins? How does it avoid mistaking different amino acids (or "letters") when forming combinations?

How does it make certain that the biochemical "language" of proteins is the same in each person?

The answer to these questions can be found in our genetic material, our genes. The nucleus of every cell contains an identical copy of the genetic substance of both the parental egg and sperm cells. Without discussing too many biochemical details it is important to point out that the formation of proteins is dictated by the genes contained in the cell's nucleus. Proteins are transcripts of the genetic code.

The proteins of our blood mainly stem from the liver cells and from certain defensive cells known as B–lymphocytes. The main protein of our blood serum—which accounts for 60 percent of all our protein—is called albumin and comes from the liver. The remaining 40 percent are subsumed under the term globulin. A measuring technique called electrophoresis uses electric current to divide globulins into alpha, beta, and gamma globulins, and alpha globulins into two further subgroups, alpha–1 and alpha–2. The alpha–2, beta, and gamma fractions of our globulins are each composed of several hundred or thousand different proteins, while albumin and alpha–1 globulin as a rule are each constituted by a single protein.

Of medical importance are mainly the alpha–2 and gamma globulins which increase during inflammation processes. Acute and sudden inflammations lead to elevated alpha–2 globulin counts, while slow chronic inflammations lead to an increase in gamma globulins.

Gamma globulins are the antibodies discussed in the first chapter. They stem from mature B–lymphocytes, called plasma cells. Their task is to identify substances that are foreign to our body or that remain after cells have died.

Alpha–2 and beta globulins are a varied mixture of proteins and are not easy to fit into some larger scheme. They are distinguished according to their function into transport proteins, inflammation proteins, tumor proteins, and others. Because we will introduce them one by one in the context of individual diseases, we will only give an initial summary here and in the following list.

*Diagnostically important blood proteins and their significance**

NAME	SIGNIFICANCE
AFP (Alpha-Feto-Protein)	Tumor marker
Albumin	Main blood protein

NAME	SIGNIFICANCE
Antibody	Immune globulin (See below.)
Antithrombin III	Anticoagulant (co-factor)
Alpha–1 Antitrypsin	Enzyme inhibitor, inflammation protein, acute phase reactant
Apolipoprotein A,B,C,D,E	Part of the lipoproteins
Autoantibodies	Immune globulins directed against substances in our own bodies
CA 125, CA 15–3	Tumor markers
CEA (Carcinoembryonic antigen)	Tumor marker
Ceruloplasmin	Copper transport protein, inflammation protein, acute phase reactant
C–reactive protein	Inflammation protein
Ferritin	Iron storage protein, inflammation protein, acute phase reactant
Fibrinogen	Immediate precursor of the blood clot inflammation protein, acute phase reactant
Globulin	Generic term for all blood proteins except albumin
Hemoglobin (not in serum)	Red blood pigment, oxygen-carrying protein
Haptoglobin	Mucoprotein to which hemoglobin is bound; inflammation protein
Immune globulin A,D,E,G,M	Defensive substances, antibody proteins
Complement C3, C4	Inflammation proteins
alpha–1, beta–2 Microglobulin	Renal function, tumor marker

NAME	SIGNIFICANCE
Myoglobin	Oxygen-binding protein related to hemoglobin in the heart and skeletal muscles
Plasminogen	Precursor of clot degrading proteins (plasmin)
Protein C, S	Inhibitors of clotting cascade
PSA (Prostate-specific antigen)	Tumor marker
Thyroglobulin	Thyroid-hormone-binding protein, tumor marker
TPA (Tissue plasminogen activator)	Promoter of clot dissolution
Transferrin	Iron transport protein, inflammation protein
Tumor marker	Generic term for various proteins that can be measured when benign or malignant tumors are present, or in case of inflammation.

(*Hormones are described in chapter 9.)

Transport proteins serve as a type of packaging for substances which in their natural state are not easily soluble in the blood, or for those that are so valuable that our body does not want them to be present in the bloodstream without protection. Included among the transport proteins are apoproteins of our lipid metabolism, ceruloplasmin, transferrin, and haptoglobin as transport agent for copper, iron and red blood pigment.

Inflammation proteins fulfill many different tasks by defending against bacteria or viruses, by destroying material from cells that have died, and in the fight against cell growths (tumors). They can be subdivided roughly into the already mentioned gamma-globulins and into a diverse group of functional proteins that are referred to by the term acute phase reactant (C–reactive protein, or CRP for short).

Tumor markers, despite a name which may not inspire confidence, are not simply "cancer proteins" as the popular press is sometimes fond of describing them. Instead, they are proteins that the mature, healthy cells in our body produce only in small amounts. As a result of various pathological changes in the cells, of which cancer is only one possibility among many, the production rate of these proteins is increased, so that they can be detected in the blood at a higher concentration. The most typical conditions leading to an increase in tumor markers are both benign and malignant forms of cell multiplication as well as inflammation. It is extremely important to keep in mind that tumor markers are not used to detect tumors and even less so for proving malignancy.

Instead, their most important use in blood testing is in the monitoring of therapeutic success in known cases of tumors, for example, after breast removal or during radiation therapy. Non-specific measuring of tumor marker levels in the hope of finding a tumor is a waste of time and money. Because of their complicated names, tumor markers are almost always referred to in lab test result sheets by acronyms or sometimes numbers (for example, CA 15–3 or CEA).

Our enzymes are another type of substance that plays a special role in blood testing. Because of their biological importance they are covered in a chapter of their own. The following list of enzymes contains information about the non-enzymatic blood proteins and their biological and medical significance.

▶ *Enzymes*

The substances known as proteins is so overwhelmingly large compared to carbohydrates or lipids, because of the function they fulfill. They are not merely the initial or final products of metabolic processes. Instead many of them actually cause these metabolic processes, they determine their direction, their speed, and they group various metabolic pathways into functional units. It is fair to say that all living cells in their variety of forms and capabilities are mainly a network of proteins that absorb all other substances (like carbohydrates, lipids, minerals, sugars, and water), like a sponge and then process them in their interiors.

During the course of this chemical processing the proteins themselves are not used up or changed fundamentally. They are like a car's catalytic converter which affects the combustion of exhaust gases and reduces their harmful components without being consumed in the process. That is why these catalytic proteins are called biocatalysts or enzymes. An older term, "ferment," is no longer being used.

Enzymes are very important in blood testing. Two areas of enzyme measurement are combined under the term enzymatic analysis. On the one hand, enzymes released by damaged cells are indicators of tissue or organ damage and can be detected directly in the blood. Enzymes are also used to measure other substances in our blood, but for this purpose they are produced in an industrial process from animal or bacterial cells.

This chapter will discuss only the determining of organ damage by measuring blood enzyme levels. As a rule, test are not designed to measure the amount of an enzyme in grams or mols, instead they measure its metabolic performance, which is called, enzyme activity. It is measured in "units" (abbreviated "U"), or in the new SI system.

Since enzymes are very sensitive in their reaction to variations in measurement conditions it is difficult to establish normal values. As with all vital processes, enzyme activity depends primarily on temperature. In most countries, enzyme measurements are conducted at body temperature (98.6°F or 37°C). However, in some countries these temperatures vary even from one lab to another so that the normal values also differ. Unfortunately a world-wide standard has not yet been established.

The enzymes in our blood and their organ sources

ABBREVIATION (NAME)	ORGAN OF ORIGIN
(Amylase)	Pancreas, parotid gland
AP; ALK.phos (Alkaline phosphatase)	Liver, bone, intestine and others
CK, CPK (Creatinekinase)	Skeletal muscles, heart
CK–MB (Creatinekinase–MB)	Heart
SGOT (=AST) (Glutamate-oxalacetate-transaminase)	Skeletal muscles, heart, liver
SGPT (=ALT) (Glutamate-pyruvate-transaminase)	Liver
gamma-GT (gamma-glutamyltranspeptidase)	Liver
LDH (Lactate-dehydrogenase)	Liver, skeletal muscles, heart, blood cells
(Lipase)	Pancreas

Enzymes are easily recognized by their names because they all share the ending "-ase" (lactate-dehydrogenase (LDH), creatinekinase (CK), glutamate-pyruvate-transaminase (GPT)). Lab test results usually only give the abbreviated names, but even then they are easily recognized by the unit of measurement, U/l (units per liter).

Since almost every enzyme that can be detected in the blood stems from damaged cells, the enzyme's activity permits the physician to draw conclusions about its origin and the affected organ. For instance, CK stems mainly from muscle cells and GPT from liver cells. The table of blood enzymes shows our most important blood enzymes and the organs they come from.

A special type of enzymes are the coagulation factors, whose task is to seal leaks in our blood circulation system. Formed in the liver in the form of inactive preliminary substances, they circulate in our blood in a holding pattern. If a blood vessel is injured the surrounding tissue releases substances into the blood which activate the dormant coagulation factors. In a complex interplay known as the coagulation cascade, active coagulation factors attack other, still inactive ones and activate them in turn. At the end of the few minutes which this process takes, the coagulation factor thrombin is activated and triggers the formation of the actual blood clot. It does this by breaking down the blood protein fibrinogen, which constitutes only 0.2 to 0.3 percent of the plasma's total weight. In its liquid state, individual fibrinogen molecules swim freely in the bloodstream without touching one another. The effect of activated thrombin is that fibrinogen forms another, slightly smaller protein, known as fibrin. The breaking down of fibrinogen into fibrin acts like removing a protective cap from a magnet: fibrin molecules now attract one another and form a spongy net whose mesh catches both solid and liquid blood components. This clot composed of fibrin and of various cells closes the blood vessel's defect and prevents us from bleeding to death.

Blood tests do not uncommonly measure individual coagulation enzymes, since coagulation is the result not of a single enzyme but of teamwork. Instead, global tests are used to measure the length of time that elapses in a test tube between the start of the activation phase and the formation of the blood clot. The more time this process takes the less effective the entire team of coagulation enzymes is.

A well-known clotting test used to be the "Quick-test," named after the American physician Armand Quick, who at the beginning of the 20th century developed a method for recognizing coagulation disorders. Tests like it, for example, usually the PT (prothrombin time)

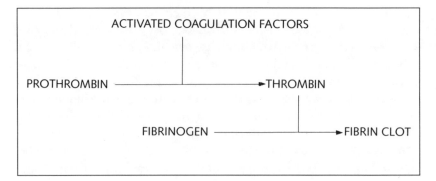

ACTIVATED COAGULATION FACTORS

PROTHROMBIN ————————————→THROMBIN

FIBRINOGEN ————————————→FIBRIN CLOT

Simplified schematic diagram of coagulation (the coagulation cascade)

test, are mainly used on patients who are being treated with anticoagulants. In patients whose blood vessels are obstructed as a result of pathological disturbances in clotting processes, the physician will use medication to lower the value to about one quarter normal in order to prevent further clots from developing. A coagulation card is used to record regularly measured clotting times, and to provide information about the artificially lowered performance of the coagulatory system. This is done so that in the event of an accident or an operation, countermeasures can be taken against excessive bleeding.

▶ *Other Measured Substances*

MINERALS   Beside the three main groups of metabolic substances, carbohydrates, lipids, and proteins, there are many other substances in our blood that can be measured and whose different levels of concentration can provide medically valuable information. Minerals are salt-like compounds that occur not only in living organisms but also in inanimate nature, such as in rock. Minerals therefore belong to the realm of "inorganic" (non-living) chemistry, in contrast to organic chemistry and biochemistry, both of which are concerned with the chemical processes in living organisms. The largest portions of the total mineral content in our blood are sodium and chloride. The compound they form, sodium chloride (table salt), is a white crystalline powder that dissolves and becomes invisible in liquids, such as water. During this process the salt divides into its two components, sodium and chloride, which in chemical language are called ions.

Other ions which occur in the blood in smaller amounts are potassium, calcium, magnesium, iron, copper, phosphate, and bicarbonate.

Usually the physician looks primarily for any deficiency in these minerals. Decreases in concentration can be caused by an insufficient diet or disturbances in the body's regulatory mechanisms, and they can cause functional disorders in certain organs.

A potassium deficiency, for example, can trigger irregularities in heart rhythm, a calcium deficiency can cause cramps, an iron deficiency can cause low energy, and a phosphate deficiency can lead to a loss of consciousness. Excessively high ion counts rarely indicate dietary imbalances and almost always stem from regulatory disorders.

HORMONES Among the list of metabolic components of our blood we should also mention hormones. They are similar to enzymes in that they help control our metabolism. The concentration of hormones in our blood is extremely small—as a rule no more than millionths of grams per liter—but they are highly effective, nonetheless.

They can bind very specifically to selected body cells and give commands to their enzymes. This "command language" of course works chemically: the binding of a hormone to a body cell causes the production of chemical messenger substances which are called "second messengers." In measuring hormone concentrations in the blood it is usually assumed that a high hormone level leads to increased effectiveness, and a low level leads to a decreased effectiveness. The most important hormones for blood testing are the thyroid hormones thyroxine and triiodothyronine (commonly abbreviated "T4" and "T3"), and the hormone TSH (thyroid-stimulating hormone) that stimulates the thyroid (Latin: glandula thyreoidea) gland to produce hormones. These hormones are described in detail in chapter 9. Other important hormones are cortisol, adrenaline, and noradrenaline from the adrenal gland, parathormon from the parathyroid gland, prolactin and growth hormone (TSH for short) from our brain, as well as the various sex hormones, progesterone, testosterone, and the various estrogens.

SUMMARY

Most of the substances that can be measured in the blood can be divided into three main groups. The carbohydrates, or sugars, and their storage and metabolic products are one group. The lipids mainly include cholesterol and triglycerides (neutral fats) which have gained great notoriety on account of the role they have been found to play in the development of heart attacks. The proteins are the most varied group of blood substances. They fulfill numerous roles in our metabolism, in defense, transportation, and many other tasks. One particularly important subgroup of blood proteins is our enzymes which control metabolic processes as biocatalysts. Beside these three main groups there are important minerals, such as potassium or iron. Hormones are a class of messenger substances, that are highly effective even in extremely low concentrations.

►► Tracking Down the Causes of Disease

The different concentrations of the substances we described in the last chapter can provide a fairly exact description of the state of our organism, as we have shown. But this does not even begin to exhaust the analytic powers of blood testing. In this and the next chapter we will show how blood testing helps us to discover the causes of certain diseases, and to make prognoses about their further course. Informally you might say: Blood values actually permit a look into the past and future of some diseases.

In medical terminology, a review of the causes and development of a disease is called etiology (from the Greek *aitia:* cause, and *logos:* science), and the prediction of its future development is called prognosis (from the Greek *prognosis:* knowing the future).

► An Example of the Study of the Causes of Disease

A twenty-year old man is taken to hospital after suffering from a severe circulatory collapse. Questioning the patient and his family, examining the blood values for heart muscle enzymes (see chapter 5), and examining the EKG lead to the diagnosis heart attack despite the patient's youth. Since infarctions are extremely rare in twenty-year-olds, the physicians are at first surprised.

► How Could This Infarct Have Developed?

During the recovery period over the next few days no new clues are uncovered, despite intensive questioning and further testing. The young man has never smoked and has generally maintained a healthy lifestyle: only moderate amounts of alcohol, a sensible diet, and regular exercise have been a normal part of his life. While the treatment is successful many questions remain unanswered. Why did the heart attack occur, and what are the possibilities for specific preventative measures against another attack?

Blood testing of the lipid (fat) metabolism finally provides a decisive clue. While triglyceride levels are within the normal range, the young man's cholesterol level is at 500 mg/dl and far higher than the average among healthy people. A more detailed examination (see p. 170) produces a low value of 20 mg/dl for the "good" HDL-cholesterol, and a severely elevated level of 440 mg/dl for the "bad" LDL-cholesterol. The LDL concentration should be less than 150 mg/dl in healthy people.

The reasons for the high LDL-cholesterol level become still clearer after sophisticated blood cell and connective tissue cell tests: The young man is suffering from a congenital deficiency of so-called LDL receptors. In testing his parents, the same deficiency is discovered, although to a lesser extent.

LDL receptors are parts of the cell membrane and are responsible for absorbing LDL-cholesterol from the blood into our body cells. A reduced number of these receptors leads to an insufficient use of LDL by the body cells and to an LDL congestion in the blood.

Two Americans, Brown and Goldstein, won the Nobel prize for clarifying the causal connection between LDL receptors and arteriosclerosis. They found that a congestion of LDL in the blood triggers the body's "police force," the macrophages. These feeding cells first gorge themselves on the LDL blood particles in order to reduce the congestion, and afterwards perish. Where they come to rest they form calcifying plaques (from the French *plaque:* plate) which, in connection with other factors, lead to a gradual occlusion of the blood vessels.

This process is not a sudden event but takes years and decades. Although some details of the process of infarction development are still unclear, the case of the young man points to one fact: The early infarction is the result of a congenital disease, namely a lack of LDL receptors which he has inherited from his parents. This deficiency can be determined by a specific blood test.

Based on an understanding of the causes, strategies can be developed for further treatment and prevention. These range from an almost cholesterol-free diet and certain medications to a sophisticated dialysis, and, of course, genetic counselling in the event that the patient plans to have children.

Detecting congenital disease is one of the most interesting tasks of blood analysis. Especially with inherited diseases that are present at birth, the future fate of the patient and his family depends on an early diagnosis, since these disorders can cause permanent damage if they go unrecognized.

A well-known and fortunately rare example is acute intermittent porphyria, a disruption in the formation of red blood pigment which is often inherited and is accompanied by sudden and severe abdominal pain. Unrecognized, the symptoms can lead to a false diagnosis of appendicitis, since the pain caused by both diseases is very similar, and since congenital porphyria is so rare as to be seldom suspected and tested for. It has happened that patients suffering from porphyria underwent surgery for their apparent appendicitis.

Unfortunately, in the long run porphyria leads to changes in the nervous system and in the patient's psyche, which may lead to a further false diagnosis such as "hysteria." In this way false readings of the symptoms can persist until specific testing leads to a diagnosis of porphyria. The first hint often comes from testing the patient's urine because it changes to a dark red color when left exposed to sunlight.

A precise diagnosis of porphyria, making a careful distinction between its many subvariants then requires the chemical analysis of blood, urine, and feces with sophisticated methods.

In the two cases, LDL receptor deficiency and porphyria, it was possible to recognize a genetic disorder by its effects, without having to examine the genetic material (the chromosomes) directly. In the first the effect was a congestion of cholesterol in the blood, and in the second it was the presence of a light sensitive pigment in the urine.

▶ *Examining the Genetic Material*

The increasing sophistication of biochemical techniques since the late 1980's has made it possible to examine genetic diseases where their actual causes lie: in the genetic material itself. As material for examination any body cell is suitable, from organs such as our skin and hair to liver or muscle cells. This is because every nucleus contains a complete, identical copy of the genetic information of both parents. In practice, blood cells have proven useful because they are easy to obtain. For genetic testing only our white blood cells, the leukocytes can be used because the other cells, erythrocytes and thrombocytes, do not contain a nucleus.

Only a small portion of human genetic information has as yet been decoded, because the so-called genetic code of human beings is extremely extensive. If we describe the genetic information about a virus as fully a typewritten page, then our human genetic code would fill the equivalent of a library containing several thousand volumes.

In the meantime, some of the genetic information that is important for medical science has been deciphered, as a result of extremely painstaking scientific labor. An example are some parts of the genetic code that are responsible for progressive muscular dystrophy. Patients with this disease suffer from a progressive weakening of the muscles which can force them to live in a wheelchair even when they are still children. After a partial decoding of our genetic information it became possible to develop so-called gene-probes for the disease. With their help it became possible to find defects in the genetic code and to make them visible. We now know that muscular dystrophy is not triggered by a single wrong "letter" in the genetic code, but that it can be triggered by a variety of changes, all of which lead to the same symptom, loss of muscle mass.

Polymerase chain reaction, or PCR, was developed only in 1985 and has become something of a catch phrase. It is an analysis technique which enables the genetic substance of single cells to be multiplied thousands and millions of times in only a few hours, therefore permitting testing for specific changes. It is used to find and diagnose not only viruses that have "sneaked" into the patient's genetic material, but also an increasing number of mutations (changes) in human genes that can make us ill.

Physicians and scientists speculate that the rapid pace at which analytic technology is developing will soon lead to an understanding of the genetic causes for common diseases like diabetes, gout, and even cancer. This process has already begun.

▶ *Investigating Infections*

Another large group of diseases that can be detected from our blood are the infectious diseases. Quite often bacteria can be cultured in a test tube, (grown in vitro) from the blood or other body fluids. In addition, foreign intruders, like bacteria and viruses leave traces in the blood serum in the form of antibodies. Here proteins which belong to the globulins are produced by specialized lymphocytes and are used to identify and quickly destroy foreign substances if they intrude in our organism again.

To ascertain whether an initially unidentified disease is or was caused by a certain bacterium or virus, the patient's serum is mixed with the suspected germ, or some of its isolated components, and examined for a reaction by the serum's antibodies. If the test is positive the serum sample is diluted in order to find out the concentration level of antibodies that have been produced to fight the germ in question. The final result of the analysis is the minimum amount of dilution at which a positive reaction can still be observed. The more concentrated the solution—the specialized term is titer (from the French *titre:* standard)—the more antibodies are present. Testing of this kind is the main task of a separate discipline within laboratory diagnostics known as serology.

These serum examinations have actually less to do with recognizing infections such as flu, fever, or diarrhea than with the diagnosis of severe and potentially life-threatening diseases. The best-known example is infectious inflammation of the liver, viral hepatitis, which can be transmitted, for example, by blood transfusions. By determining the titer pattern one can know whether an infection has taken place, whether the disease is new or whether it has been present for some time, and whether the patient's blood is still infectious. This is discussed in more detail in chapter 6.

Many other virus infections such as AIDS, Pfeiffer's glandular fever, and German measles can be detected in a similar fashion. Titer examinations are also useful in diagnosing some bacterial infections and deep-seated fungus infections in patients whose immune system is weakened. Invasions of the inner organs by parasites, such as the canine tape worm, *Echinococcus,* which leaves behind liquid-filled cavities in the liver and lungs, also leave behind a detectable antibody titer.

The spectrum of diseases that can be recognized with the help of blood tests far exceeds the genetic diseases and infections we have mentioned. The reason those two categories have been discussed in more detail is that their causes are known. For most other sicknesses—apart from accidents and poisoning—medical science has still not found a definitive etiology.

Such complaints as the large group of rheumatic pains have been researched only partially for their causes. Consequently they cannot be recognized in the blood with any certainty. For these cases we have only examination techniques that point towards some possible causes without proving any of them. For example, many patients who suffer from rheumatism carry antibodies against their own body-tissue. It seems that these are cases of a misguided defensive reaction of the body against itself. However, the actual reason why the body produces defensive substances against its own cells, and why these antibodies trigger pain in some patients and not in others is still unknown.

SUMMARY

Blood tests not only permit diseases to be recognized and described but often also give clues as to their causes. If a disease has genetic causes it is usually possible both to determine the effect of the genetic disturbance in the blood, and to examine the genetic material itself. If on the other hand a disease is caused by foreign organisms, such as viruses, these can be detected by analyzing the antibodies present in the blood. The causes for numerous diseases are still unknown, and they cannot be detected via blood testing.

▸▸ *Prognoses*

As well as determining the causes of a pathological process before it has broken out fully, by using a blood test, it is also possible to predict roughly when the first complaints may occur, and what course the disease will take if it is left untreated. A distinction must be made between those blood analyses that discover the actual causes of disease, like changes in our genetic material, and those that can predict its future course based on its early symptoms. But in both cases, the fact is that 100 percent certainty in predicting sickness is as impossible as it is in predicting the weather.

Using the example of genetic diseases again, since our genetic material is almost completely determined at the time of conception we can recognize such pathological changes as defective chromosomes or genes very early and often even before birth. This means that with the specific use of diagnostic tests it is possible to act early and possibly avoid severe consequences. Medical clinics that have specialized in this type of problem provide what is known as genetic counselling.

Especially couples who are genetically at risk and who want to have children should consider asking for the advice of a specialist.

The increasing sophistication of our analytic techniques may one day make it possible to recognize not only rare and severe diseases, such as muscular dystrophy before they have developed, but also the more common disorders, such as diabetes. Even a tendency for developing cancer given certain, strictly defined environmental factors, is beginning to be predictable from the genetic material.

▶ *Prognostic Markers*

The blood tests which allow a "look into the future" involve blood components which do not trigger any diseases themselves, and do not even indicate any carriers of disease directly. Instead they contain information about the severity of a disease, and thus indirectly about its future course and possible outcome.

Blood components whose measurement permits such predictions are known as "prognostic markers." This is still a relatively new area of medicine but it is developing rapidly. To forestall any exaggerated expectations we should begin by pointing out that these markers do not allow for absolute certainty in predicting the development of a disease. At most they can indicate a probability for a more or less positive development. (A hurricane may also move in an unexpected direction, despite our best efforts at monitoring and prediction!)

These prognostic methods are of great interest for the treatment of patients after a traffic accident or a severe operation. Their fate depends on many individual factors, such as type and severity of trauma or operation, as well as the age and general condition of the patient. Some people survive extremely severe accidents while others die from comparatively minor injuries.

Since these patients are often unconscious for days while their vital functions are being maintained by machines, to judge a patient's condition physicians depend on test results from the regular monitoring of temperature, blood pressure, and blood values. These combined findings usually permit an assessment of the healing process, even when a patient cannot be asked directly.

Among the different blood tests we distinguish between those that indicate the location of a disease, as in kidney failure, and those that indicate "severity." The former are known as organ markers, and the latter are called prognostic markers.

These markers are substances from our body's defensive system, mostly proteins from the liver and from the blood cells. C−reactive protein (CRP for short) is one such example, and has been particularly well studied. High measured values of this substance indicate that the organism has to perform at a high level of defensive activity and that it is consequently more at risk.

At the beginning of a severe disease, like immediately after a car accident that has caused a large number of bone fractures and organ injuries, the defensive substance CRP is always present in the blood at high levels of concentration. During a normal process of recovery the measured value decreases within a few days. If complications occur it increases or at least remains elevated. Generally, an elevated level of CRP indicates complications in the healing process and prompts the physician to conduct a concentrated search for possible causes.

Even illnesses that are not the result of an external force are often difficult to predict in their development. A well-known example is acute pancreatitis which is a sudden inflammation of the pancreas. It seems to come "out of the blue" and often after consuming alcohol or a rich meal. Patients suffer from extremely severe abdominal pain which requires immediate hospitalization. Once there, an inflammation of the pancreas is easily detected with the help of a blood test. Amylase and lipase, the two organ markers will have strongly increased values, but these will not reveal whether the patient will be able to leave the hospital after a few days in perfect health, or whether severe, and in extreme cases, even deadly complications will soon develop.

However, measuring the levels of these prognostic markers is useful in assessing the severity of the disease. If the measured values remain normal or if they normalize in a short time, it means that spontaneous healing can be expected which may only need some support by special diet and medication. If, on the other hand, these values increase strongly a severe form of pancreatitis is very likely which may necessitate a quick surgical procedure.

The detection of prognostic markers is still in its infancy. To determine the individual risk factors in a severely ill patient these laboratory values alone are insufficient. The physician needs other clinical information about the course of the disease, and most of all, a lot of experience, in order to give an even approximately accurate estimation of the patient's fate.

SUMMARY

Medical science is increasingly attempting to use blood tests to predict the future development of diseases. In genetic disorders and with hidden inflammations early testing allows countermeasures to be taken even before severe symptoms of the disease have appeared. For diseases whose course is unpredictable, prognostic markers are used in an attempt to predict, and if possible, prevent complications.

►► *Medications and Poisons*

In looking at the causes and effects of disease we must also discuss medications and poisons. They influence the course of a disease in decisive ways, and they can even by its original cause. Using the methods of modern analysis it is possible to detect amounts as low as millionths of a gram of foreign substances in the blood and in other body fluids.

These measurements are used either to determine whether a certain substance is present at all in the blood, or else to find its concentration and determine if there has been an overdose. The first case is known as qualitative and the second as quantitative analysis.

A purely qualitative analysis is usually sufficient for detecting poisons. Whether the substance is a drug, such as hashish or heroin, or a poisonous compound, like arsenic or cyanide, or medication taken in order to commit suicide a positive finding will result in countermeasures such as gastric irrigation, or dialysis, and in increased supervision of the patient.

When a medication has been given in the course of treating a disease, the qualitative analysis should always be positive—unless the patient has not taken the medicine, which unfortunately sometimes has to be controlled by chemical analysis, as well. The physician must determine the exact concentration of the medication in the blood or in the body fluids that the medication will be effective for healing. With most medications the patient need only follow exactly the manufacturer's or the physician's instructions in order to make sure that there is an effective concentration in the body. But with some medications this rule does not hold. These are mostly highly potent substances that can produce undesirable side-effects when present in very high concentrations, and which fail to be effective in very low ones. The term used to describe this phenomenon is the "therapeutic range" of a drug.

A wide therapeutic range means that there is a large difference between dosages that are still barely effective and those that are dangerously high. In these cases a quantitative analysis is usually unnecessary. A narrow therapeutic range, on the other hand, means that giving the drug to a patient can mean walking a tightrope between insufficient effectiveness and undesirable side-effects. Here monitoring of the drug's level in the blood is recommended.

As well as the quantitative analysis of medications as part of therapeutic monitoring, it may sometimes be necessary to measure the exact concentration of a poison. This happens where a foreign substance is harmless in small quantities but poisonous in large concentrations. For example, alcohol has a stimulating effect on most people when they consume small quantities, but in large doses it can lead to loss of consciousness and death. A similar situation exists with metals, such as iron, copper, cadmium, and lead, and of course with the abuse of prescribed drugs. Benzodiazepine, for example, can be taken in low doses as a sedative without any danger, but high concentrations can suppress breathing and cause death.

► *Alcohol—A Stimulating Poison*

Because of its enormous impact as a stimulant, we will treat alcohol in more depth in the following chapter.

If alcohol was less dangerous to health it could be looked upon as an almost ideal energy source since it is liquid, universally usable, tastes good, and has the highest energy content after fat. However it lacks minerals, proteins, and vitamins.

The consequences of excessive alcohol consumption to physical and mental health are terrible. Long, continuous abuse of alcohol damages nearly every organ in the human body, but in particular the liver and the nervous system. Since this damage affects also the brain, and with it the central switching station of the nervous system, the alcoholic's psyche and social environment are also affected. According to expert estimates alcohol threatens the existence of every tenth family. In the U.S.A., 10 percent of men and 3 to 5 percent of women are considered alcoholics.

Blood alcohol level testing is not used to monitor chronic patients, but instead, for those who suffer from acute (short-lived) disruptions of consciousness. Most often alcohol content is measured when patients suffering from disturbance of consciousness are admitted to a hospital, or in connection with driving offenses. The physician is mainly interested in distinguishing those who are "merely drunk" from those who have consumed drugs or medication as well, or those whose consciousness is clouded by metabolic disorders or other diseases. Since alcohol is often consumed together with barbiturates, sedatives, or other drugs, a large number of sophisticated blood tests, as well as urine tests are often needed to determine the reasons for an unclear disturbance of consciousness.

There is only a loose connection between the concentration of alcohol in a person's blood and the externally recognizable signs. Someone who has never before consumed alcohol can appear drunk at no more than 0.2 to 0.3 g/l, while alcoholics who can "hold their liquor" frequently show no sign of being affected at even 2 or 3 g/l. The lowest blood alcohol concentrations that can be measured, using an acceptable expenditure of time and money, are 0.1 to 0.2 g/l, while the highest recorded values that have been survived were about 6 g/l of blood and 7.5 g/l of serum.

Approximate clinical values for determining blood alcohol levels

BLOOD CONCENTRATION	STATE	BEHAVIORAL INDICATORS
0–0.5 g/l	sober	
0.5–1.5 g/l	slightly drunk	talkative, lack of judgement, animated mood
1.5–2.5 g/l	drunk	vision and balance affected, loss of depth perception
2.5–3.5 g/l	very drunk	loss of motor control, slurred speech, confusion
above 3.5 g/l	alcohol poisoning	disrupted breathing, progressive depression of consciousness, loss of reflexes

The difference between measurements in blood and serum is due to the fact that alcohol concentration is lower in the blood cells than in the surrounding blood liquid. The limit of 0.8 g/l which is important in traffic offenses is measured in blood. Usually, hospitals use serum levels internally and indicate blood concentrations for legal purposes. The difference between the two values is about 20 percent.

The importance of determining exact alcohol levels in order to avoid errors in judgement was confirmed by evaluations of 5,000 blood tests ordered by the police. In every sixth case with blood alcohol levels between 2.5 and 3 g/l the physician taking the sample suspected no or very little alcohol. The figures in the Blood Concentration table help to explain how average blood alcohol concentrations are determined in normal persons.

It is also useful to know how quickly blood alcohol levels decrease. Here we find strong individual variations that are determined by gender, race, and other genetic factors. Very generally we can say that every hour 0.1 to 0.2 g/l of alcohol are removed from the blood. If immediately after drinking 1.05 pints (.5 liter) of wine a person's blood alcohol level is 1.0 g/l, then it will take 5 to 10 hours for the alcohol to be completely metabolized. If the level is 2.0 g/l, which is usually accompanied by a definite feeling of drunkenness, the remaining alcohol concentration may be as high as 1 g/l even after 8 hours of sleep.

The computing of blood alcohol levels from breath tests is virtually impossible. The well-known "Breathalyzer" tests used by the police in traffic checks can give only a rough indication of the degree of alcoholization. They are not suitable for legal purposes, because there are too many other possibly disruptive influences at play.

SUMMARY

Determining the presence and level of foreign substances in our blood is becoming increasingly important in medical science. For the analysis of poisons, a qualitative analysis of whether or not a substance is present is usually enough. But the measurement of medications requires a quantitative analysis of the level of concentration, in order to recognize, for example, excessively large or small doses. Blood alcohol levels are mainly measured to determine the cause of disturbances of consciousness, or to establish legal driving limits. Values higher than 3.5 g/l usually indicate alcohol poisoning.

➤➤ *The So-Called Laboratory Diseases*

The last chapter of this part of the book is about a number of diseases which strictly speaking do not exist: the so-called laboratory diseases. They are important because, by causing blood values outside the normal range, they can mimic certain other diseases. This in turn may mean that a patient is diagnosed with a disease that is not actually present, and that either the wrong therapeutic measures are taken, or that an actual disease is overlooked.

The best-known example of such a laboratory disease is macro-amylasemia. In this variation on normal blood values, a special form of amylase is present. In the section on enzymes, amylase was described as a marker substance for diseases of the pancreas. Amylase is a small enzyme molecule that is normally quickly flushed out by the kidneys and as a result does not usually appear in large amounts in our blood. Patients suffering from macroamylasemia have a particular form of amylase which is bound to an immune globulin, and because of the increase in size the molecules can no longer be flushed out by the kidneys. They are metabolized very slowly by the body, and are detectable in persistently high blood concentrations.

By itself a high amylase concentration has no negative consequences for the carriers of macroamylasemia. But things can become quite unpleasant for someone with macroamylasemia if their laboratory disease has not been detected before, and if they happen to see a physician—for example during an intestinal infection—because of abdominal pain. The physician will measure amylase as part of the blood test, and because of the high levels a wrong suspicion can easily arise. At first, the physician may suspect pancreatitis (inflammation of the pancreas). It takes a great deal of experience for the physician to exclude the wrong diagnosis based on the harmless increase in amylase and find the true cause of the abdominal pain.

One way to avoid being lured on the wrong track by macroamylasemia is to measure a second pancreatic enzyme beside amylase at the same time, for example, lipase. Only if both enzymes are elevated do the findings point towards pancreatitis. Another solution is to additionally measure the so-called p—amylase (p here indicates pancreatic) with the help of a special immune test which does not react to the macroenzyme, or to determine enzyme molecule size in a specialized laboratory. Also, a physical examination and identifying typical pain symptoms will allow the physician to distinguish between pancreatitis and other causes of abdominal pain, such as intestinal infections.

The diagnosis of another laboratory disease is just as problematic. It involves a giant enzyme, creatinekinase (CK) that is typical in coronary infarctions. Here enlarged enzyme molecules cause a seemingly pathological increase in creatinekinase blood values. And again, the physician can be led astray—for example, if a patient also complains of chest pains. Since macro-creatinekinase, like a heart attack appears mainly in older persons, the carrier of a macro-CK may possibly at first be treated for a heart attack despite the fact that the chest pains are in fact caused by degenerative symptoms of the spine.

Again, there are ways of distinguishing between true and apparent heart attacks. Physical examination, questioning the patient, performing an EKG, and a series of special examinations usually lead to the correct diagnosis. Once a diagnosis of laboratory disease has been ascertained, carriers of macro-CK will no longer have to undergo complicated additional tests.

Occasionally, laboratory disease also refers to cases in which individual blood values are slightly outside of the normal range. As normal ranges include not 100 percent but only 95 percent of all healthy persons, every twentieth healthy person will have some blood values that exceed these ranges. An experienced physician will check these values and consider other findings, before making a premature diagnosis and declaring a healthy person to be suffering a laboratory disease.

SUMMARY

Blood tests can occasionally mimic nonexistent diseases which are known as laboratory diseases. In most cases they turn out to be variations in the norm of certain blood components. Carriers of such variations should be informed about their special status in order to avoid being victims of wrong diagnoses.

4

THE BLOOD PICTURE OR
HEMOGRAM

►► *How Blood Components Function*

► *Blood Pigment (Hemoglobin)*

In medicine, blood is considered a self-contained organ just like our heart or liver. By using different stains an image of our blood, a blood picture, can be seen under a microscope. By counting and identifying the blood's components, which are mostly cells, and by recognizing healthy or abnormal cell forms, we can draw conclusions about changes in the blood itself and in other organs. For this reason a blood picture is always one of the most important indicators of this organ we call blood, giving us important information about our whole organism.

Blood is made up of both solid and liquid components. The liquid component is the blood plasma, while the solid part is made up of blood cells. The most numerous among our blood cells are the red blood corpuscles. They carry the red blood pigment, hemoglobin, which is responsible for our blood's red color. Its role is to transport oxygen in the body.

Bright-red blood is rich in oxygen while blue-red blood contains little oxygen. If we bleed from a wound and the color is bright red, we are seeing arterial or oxygenated blood. The different color is due to a change in the hemoglobin molecule caused by the oxygen it carries. Upon releasing oxygen blood takes on a blue-red color. Since oxygen-rich blood flows in the arteries and oxygen-starved blood flows in the veins, blood color makes it possible to tell if bleeding is arterial or venous.

▶ *Our Red Blood Corpuscles are Very Special Cells*

A single microliter (one millionth of a liter) of blood will on average contain five million red blood corpuscles, called erythrocytes. In adults these are formed in the bone marrow. They come in a variety of forms which develop from a common mother cell (stem cell), and mature in the bone marrow. When they migrate from the marrow into the bloodstream they lose their nucleus. This makes them unique among our cells, because normally all cells possess a nucleus. Having lost their nuclei the red blood cells are adapted to the peculiarities of capillary circulation. They can squeeze into the narrowest blood vessels, and this way reach every cranny of our organs in order to supply their tissue with oxygen.

There are also small numbers of preliminary cell forms of erythrocytes in the blood. Certain methods of staining them show that they have a net-like internal structure. This is why they are called reticulocytes (from the Latin *reticulum:* net).

▶ *White Blood Corpuscles—A Part of the Blood's Police Force*

Our blood contains two distinctive types of white blood corpuscles: larger ones with a variety of differently-shaped nuclei that when stained are easy to observe under a microscope, and smaller ones which tend to have uniform nucleus structures. White blood corpuscles are called leukocytes (from the Greek *leukos:* white). Some are formed in the bone marrow and are called granulocytes, some in the lymph nodes and the spleen. The latter are called lymphocytes.

According to the different shapes and granules they contain, leukocytes are divided into granulocytes and monocytes. In granulocytes the nucleus appears segmented and various types of granules are seen. If granules appear light blue the cells are called neutrophils; they are increased in bacterial infections. If granulocytes can be stained orange-red they are called eosinophils. They often appear in acute allergic reactions or in parasitic worm infections. If the granules appear a deep blue, the cells are called basophils.

Another group of leukocytes can be distinguished under the microscope: they are our monocytes. Only in recent years has their function come to be understood at least partially. They play an important role in our immunological identity, and during the later stages of the body's defense reaction. They can transform themselves into different cells, which then act as fundamental structures for the formation of scar tissue during the healing phase of infections.

LYMPHOCYTES—OUR BODY'S IDENTITY On their membranes lymphocytes carry characteristic "docking ports" which help our body to recognize its own tissues. Most lymphocytes remain in the lymph nodes and in the spleen.

The lymphatic system (lymphocytes, lymph nodes, spleen) matures as a consequence of genetic information and of encounters with foreign substances. Children's lymphatic systems are immature in certain ways because they need to encounter external influences, such as viral infections, in order to fully mature. During the first years of our lives, our body tissue's genetically based identity has not yet been established in the lymphocytes. This is why organ transplants can be carried out in children with a much lower risk of rejection.

Our lymphocytes' ability to distinguish between our own and alien tissue as a result of maturation makes them the most important cells in our cell-based immunity system. Their function has become even more important since the advent of organ transplants from foreign donors. Thus, in order to ensure the success of a transplant, the body's immune system must be deliberately weakened.

THE BLOOD SMEAR—THE ART OF LOOKING AT LEUKOCYTES We can recognize different forms of leukocytes by staining and examining them under a microscope. But it takes a great deal of experience to distinguish between their various forms.

In order to make leukocytes easily visible, a blood smear has to be prepared on a glass slide. The distribution of the various subgroups of leukocytes is described as a percentage of the total number of white blood corpuscles. The largest share is formed by granulocytic leukocytes at 60 to 70 percent, and by lymphocytes at 20 to 30 percent. All other forms constitute only a few percentage points. If there are changes in numbers or in the cells' shape, the blood smear provides an excellent image of these changes.

▶ *Blood Platelets—At the Center of the Blood Clot*

Our blood platelets (thrombocytes) also have the role of closing any injuries in the blood vessels. They accomplish this by forming a blood clot (thrombus).

A microliter of blood contains several hundred thousand blood platelets. In a modern laboratory's counting machine their number can be quickly ascertained. Determining the thrombocyte count is part of any comprehensive blood picture.

Thrombocytes play an important role in clotting and in the development of atherosclerosis of the blood vessels. This latter aspect has made them an object of more research than their primary function of sealing blood vessels following an injury.

An increased thrombocyte count (more than 1 million per microliter of blood) constitutes a significant risk of thrombosis (a major blood clot). Such levels are, however, found only where the preliminary form of thrombocytes, the megakaryocytes, are diseased. If the spleen is lost, for example, as a result of severe injuries to the upper left abdomen due to a car accident, an increase in thrombocytes can result which may lead to a serious tendency towards thrombosis.

Abnormally low thrombocyte counts of less than 80,000 per microliter can indicate that the body is consuming thrombocytes. In cases of severe bacterial infections (sepsis), or more rarely after viral infections, thrombocytes in the blood will be destroyed in greater numbers than even an increased production in the bone marrow can compensate for.

SUMMARY

A characteristic aspect of the blood picture is its red color, due to the red blood pigment hemoglobin. The building blocks of the blood picture are the blood cells. Beside the red blood corpuscles (erythrocytes) which provide oxygen transportation, the blood picture contains white blood corpuscles (leukocytes) which are divided into granulocytes, monocytes and lymphocytes. Leukocytes act as our body's defense, while another group of blood cells, the platelets (thrombocytes) are responsible for blood clotting. They also play an important role in atherosclerosis.

▸▸ *Anemia Has Many Causes*

▸ *Deficiencies in Red Blood Cells and/or Hemoglobin*

Red blood cells (erythrocytes) can be counted under a microscope. In modern labs this work is done by machines which can, at the same time, measure the amount of red blood pigment (hemoglobin) in the blood. In men, a normal blood count contains about 5 million erythrocytes per microliter and 15 grams of hemoglobin in 100 milliliters of blood. Women have slightly lower values due to their regular blood loss during menstruation. They average 4 million erythrocytes and 13 grams of hemoglobin.

▸ *Diseases of the Bone Marrow and the Destruction of Red Blood Cells*

Our blood is formed in the bone marrow. If it is affected by an illness it can no longer produce a sufficient number of red blood cells and stops inserting hemoglobin into the erythrocytes.

Because erythrocytes live approximately four months, their number gradually declines over this period of time, causing the body to develop anemia. A bone marrow test will show either an absence of bone-forming cells or a flooding of the bone marrow with alien (not bone marrow specific) cells which displace blood formation. If these cells are indeed alien to the bone marrow, they usually stem from a tumor in another organ or from the lymphatic glands. In such cases we speak of an infiltration of the bone marrow by tumor cells, as distinct from localized tumor cell nests in the bone which can lead to the destruction of the bone itself (bone metastases).

MARROW ASPIRATION—AN IMPORTANT EXAMINATION To determine if the bone marrow is diseased, a marrow sample is taken, usually from the ridge of the hip bone (iliac crest) to prepare sections (slices) and smears. Portions of the bone marrow specimen are spread on a glass slide and examined under a microscope after being stained in a particular way. This method allows an examination of specific marrow cells; sections are examined for cellularity, infiltrations, and cellular details.

Under healthy conditions there is a distinction between mature blood cells and mother cells which are found in the bone marrow. White and red blood cells, as well as platelets, share common mother cells which mature in the marrow into the preliminary cell forms of erythrocytes, leukocytes, and platelets. These preliminary cells normally do not leave the bone marrow. But during severe cases of inflammation, or anemia, the regenerative ability of the bone marrow can produce new cells in such large numbers that even preliminary cells may find their way into the bloodstream.

To distinguish whether this has been caused by an adaptation to a change in the body—inflammation or blood loss—or by an actual disease of the bone marrow, the marrow itself must be examined.

BONE MARROW DAMAGE AND TOXINS   Of all our cells bone marrow cells have the greatest ability to regenerate. New formation of red and white blood cells is constantly taking place, because even under normal conditions leukocytes have a life expectancy of no more than a few days, and erythrocytes of a few months, at most. Thrombocytes also have to be constantly regenerated, because their life expectancy is about the same as that of erythrocytes.

Because of its powerful ability to form new cells our bone marrow is very susceptible to damaging influences. Poisonous substances, including alcohol, have toxic effects on the bone marrow. Various medications also have an inhibiting effect on the marrow's cell formation. Cytostatic drugs which are used in cancer therapy have the most strongly inhibiting effect on the formation of leukocytes and thrombocytes. In unfavorable cases a complete loss of new cell formation in the bone marrow can occur. This is known as aplastic anemia, and means that in addition to the anemia, there is a reduction in the number of leukocytes and thrombocytes and their precursors. This leads to frequent infections, and to spontaneous hemorrhaging into the skin, the mucous membrances, and the urine. So as to counteract these effects in time, patients who are being treated with cytostatic drugs are monitored by frequent lab testing of their blood count.

WHEN BLOOD DISSOLVES—HEMOLYSIS   Our red blood cells carry the hemoglobin, the red blood pigment. Red blood cell membranes can be destroyed by medication, by toxins, or by changes in our immune defense system. If red blood cells are destroyed hemolysis occurs. The hemoglobin which is released into the blood is quickly broken down into bilirubin. Since the liver has only a limited capacity for releasing bilirubin into the bile, an excess of bilirubin will color the blood yellow (a symptom called "icterus"), and the patient may also become yellow or jaundiced.

▶ *Blood Lab Test for Anemia*

The sum total of all blood cells determines the amount of blood solids. The red portion of the red blood cells is called the hematocrit. It is expressed as a percentage of total blood volume. The normal value is about 45 percent.

Anemia occurs when either the hemoglobin content of the blood or the number or volume of red blood cells is significantly reduced. This reduction in hemoglobin red cell count, or hematocrit or all three measures is the laboratory sign of anemia. The automatic counting machines mentioned earlier can also measure the size and volume of erythrocytes. According to the distribution curve, the normal erythrocyte volume or mean corpuscular volume (MCV) is about 90 micrometers.

In cases of abnormally small blood cell volume (microcytic anemia), iron deficiency is often the cause, due to a disturbance in our ability to absorb iron or to chronic blood loss. With the latter, the physician will look for sources of hemorrhaging in the stomach, and the small or large intestine. Frequently the cause is an ulcer (ulcus ventriculi) or an intestinal polyp. In some cases cancer of the large intestine may also be the cause. A decreased amount of blood iron can also be detected by simple lab tests (serum iron; ferritin); more rarely, iron is given and blood iron levels are measured before and after ingestion (iron absorption test), to determine if there is a disruption in the body's ability to absorb iron.

LAB TEST FOR ANEMIA

Hemoglobin
Erythrocyte count
Erythrocyte volume
Hematrocrit
Iron
Vitamin B 12
Folic acid
Bilirubin
Reticulocytes

In cases of macrocytic anemia (abnormally large erythrocytes) the disruption in the blood cells' maturation is often caused by vitamin deficiencies. Tests will often show a deficiency in vitamin B 12 or folic acid. The levels at which both these vitamins are present in the blood can be determined by a lab test.

SUMMARY

Anemia is a reduction in hemoglobin and hematocrit measured with laboratory chemistry. Its causes are numerous. They can include insufficient cell production in the bone marrow in cases of diseases of the bone marrow, or increased destruction of erythrocytes, for example by hemolysis. It is necessary in all such cases to examine the blood count. In most cases the bone marrow must be examined as well. In addition it is advisable to determine the levels of iron, folic acid, and vitamin B 12.

►► *Inflammation—Our Body's Defensive Strategy*

Inflammation is the reaction which medicine has known the longest and studied the most. The typical signs of inflammation are pain (dolor), heat (calor), redness (rubor), swelling (tumor), and disordered function (functio laesa).

Everyone is familiar with these symptoms. The site of the inflammation is painful, it is reddish, and in many cases function is affected. If the legs are inflamed, for example, it is difficult or impossible to walk. These visible signs of inflammation are the result of complicated defensive processes in our body. Although there are no visible signs for the blood, this is, in fact, the ground on which this battle is waged.

In order to defend against bacteria or toxins, the integrity of our skin is the most important barrier. But those organs that possess mucous membranes—our intestine, mouth, ureter, bladder, and genitals, have important defensive roles as well. As long as the surface of our skin is intact it forms an effective protective barrier against intruders. In contrast to the mucous membranes, skin possesses a number of layers for protection against the environment. In mucous membranes our blood and the environment come into much closer contact, and here the blood's defensive mechanisms can be mobilized much more quickly (which explains why inflammations of the mucous membranes make themselves felt very quickly).

► *Our Defenses*

Our blood possesses many different means of defending against unwanted intruders. Its defenses are divided into the defensive substances in the blood plasma, the humoral defenses (from the Latin *humor:* liquid), and the defense by the blood cells (the cellular defense). As we have mentioned, all our leukocytes take part in the body's defense.

If a foreign body (antigen), for example a virus, enters the bloodstream it triggers a cascading defensive process that culminates in the destruction of the intruder. First the lymphocytes, carriers of our immune identity, recognize the presence of an antigen in the bloodstream. Using certain substances (interferon, interleukin), they signal to other cells to produce defensive substances (antibodies), which in turn attach themselves to the antigen and form an antigen-antibody-complex. This combination activates certain substances in the blood plasma which actively attract leukocytes, whose surface then binds the antigen-antibody-complex. Finally, the leukocyte will absorb either the entire complex or its antigen component. Specialized enzyme systems in the cell then kill the foreign body. In this process the leukocytes themselves are often destroyed as well. Waste products from their disintegration stimulate monocytes, a leukocyte subgroup, to absorb them. These acts of disposal are the source of such curative processes as scarring.

These activities are constantly taking place in our bodies, because we are never completely isolated from our environment. Minute injuries constantly admit germs into our bloodstream, our mucous membranes come into contact with airborne germs or those transmitted by physical contact, and yet we do not get sick. These defensive mechanisms create a balance between aggressive and defensive factors, and as long as this balance is being maintained we feel healthy.

SICKNESS—A DISTURBANCE IN THE EQUILIBRIUM BETWEEN AGGRESSION AND DEFENSE We get sick when our body's defenses are either overrun by too many intruders, or when they are weakened to begin with. The likelihood of contracting an infectious disease is directly proportional to the number of carriers that are present. This discovery is well-known from the development of epidemics. In order to produce an outbreak of cholera, for example, a minimum number of other disease carriers must be present besides the cholera germ. At other times small quantities of a germ will suffice to make a person sick. But in these cases the body's defense system is often weakened already (known as an immune defect).

A lot of work has gone into recognizing the factors affecting our immune system. Among others, psychological and hormonal influences play an important role; they are called immunomodulators. Great efforts are being made to identify them in the hope that these findings will improve the chances of treating malignant tumors.

INOCULATION—A CALCULATED INFLAMMATION A good example of the equilibrium between aggressive and defensive factors is seen with active inoculations. This involves introducing antigens into the bloodstream—antigens which are either reduced in their aggressivity (virulence), or so limited in number that our body's defenses can overcome the germ.

As a result, the disease will not break out, but our lymphocytes will have produced antibodies against the germ. As long as this information is contained in the lymphocytes our body will be able to produce the appropriate antibodies when confronted with the same germ. This process is the basis of all active inoculations. As the information in the cells is lost over time, the protective effect of the inoculation diminishes, and a booster becomes necessary.

In passive inoculations, antibodies from an immunized donor are injected directly. Since these will be absorbed by the body in a matter of weeks or months, such protection does not last as long as with active inoculation.

▶ Blood Lab Test for Inflammation

Inflammations cause typical changes in blood test results and in the blood picture. The blood test shows a typical inflammatory constellation. The most important tests are blood sedimentation and blood count, followed by other tests, such as C—reactive protein (CRP). By themselves these tests cannot reveal the cause of the inflammation. Thus a second series of specialized tests has to be conducted after the basic lab test is completed.

For certain constellations, lab tests can help distinguish between acute and chronic inflammations.

BLOOD SEDIMENTATION Blood sedimentation is the oldest and

best-known method of diagnosing an inflammation or infection. It is based on the speed at which solid blood components (mainly red blood cells) settle in the blood plasma, and is determined by the sedimentation rate, measured in millimeters per hour. Blood sedimentation cannot provide specific information about the cause of an inflammation and will, for example, also be affected by the presence of a tumor.

The sedimentation rate depends on changes in the blood plasma. Inflammations—but also tumors—lead to changes in the plasma which affect the sedimentation rate. Generally they cause an increase in the speed of sedimentation. Extreme sedimentation rates (100 millimeters and more during the first hour are usually caused by spreading metastasizing) tumors, or severe, chronic inflammations.

A slow sedimentation rate is found when there is an increase in cellular blood components. In these cases the hematocrit is often increased.

Normal values differ among age ranges and genders. For women and people over the age of 65, normal values are increased by 10 to 15 millimeters per hour.

THE BLOOD PICTURE (BLOOD COUNT) As soon as our white blood corpuscles enter into a defensive struggle they begin to reproduce. Thus the number of leukocytes in the blood increases. Normal values for the number of leukocytes are less than 10,000 per microliter. During acute infections these values can reach 30,000 and more. At the same time a differential blood count will show a changed distribution of subgroups. The increased leukocyte production leads to protocells being washed from the bone marrow into the bloodstream. In most cases of bacterial infection one can find a ten- to twenty-fold increase in neutrophilic granulocytic leukocytes. Virus infections often lead to an increase in lymphocytes. If the inflammation is allergic in nature, the number of eosinophilic granulocytes also increases.

In rare cases, the number and virulence of the carriers is so great that the number of leukocytes present in the body is not sufficient to fight off the disease. The result will be a drop in the number of leukocytes. Only a differential blood picture will be able to show the bone marrow's efforts to produce a sufficient number of defensive leukocytes. Changes of this type usually indicate extremely severe infections (sepsis).

ELECTROPHORESIS Blood plasma components can be divided into subgroups. The process of separation and its depiction in the shape of a distribution curve is known as electrophoresis. During an infection, two components will increase: the amount of alpha–2 globulin and of gamma globulin. While acute infections always lead to an increase in alpha–2 globulin, chronic infections also lead to an increase in gamma globulin.

HUMORAL DEFENSIVE SUBSTANCES Beside determining the presence of defensive cells, lab tests can also detect substances of our body's humoral defenses.

Frequently C–reactive protein is used as a quantitative indicator of the humoral reaction to an inflammation. Certain subgroups of the complement system and other proteins of the so-called acute phase protein system also have to be measured in order to determine the progression of an inflammation process.

An important group of inflammatory diseases not directly related to the presence of germs are the autoimmune diseases. They occur when our immune system falsely recognizes our own tissue as foreign, and triggers an immune reaction against it. In the end our immune system destroys our own body. This mechanism is at the root of chronic rheumatoid arthritis of the joints. The laboratory test procedures required to recognize this process involve a great number of autoantibody tests and are restricted to specialized laboratories. We cannot recognize autoimmune diseases from basic lab tests alone.

SUMMARY

Inflammations are the visible forms of our body's defensive processes. Lab tests such as sedimentation rate and blood count combined with electrophoresis and inflammation proteins demonstrate inflammatory processes. Symptoms such as redness, pain, and disordered function can also occur. Laboratory tests can demonstrate inflammations and their causes only in connection with clinical findings and further tests. Basic tests alone are not sufficient to diagnose inflammations.

►► *Leukemia: Cancer of the Blood*

The term leukemia describes a number of malignant blood cell diseases. Our bone marrow forms a wide range of cell types, and each of these can develop into a leukemic disease. The disease is classified according to the dominant cell type from which it developed, for example, eosinophilic leukemia which develops from precursors of the eosinophilic granulocytes. The most common and important forms of leukemia develop from the protocells of white blood corpuscles, or granulocytes, resulting in myelomonocytic leukemia, and from lymphocytes, resulting in lymphocytic leukemia. They appear in both acute and chronic forms.

▶ *Why Leukemia is a Cancer*

Cancer cells develop into a tumorous growth in the affected organ. The tumor destroys the organ because its uncontrolled growth leads to replacement of normal tissue and to loss of the organ's function. Finally, the tumor will reach the organ's boundary, and spread to other organs, either directly, by growing into them, or by sending out tumor cells through the bloodstream or the lymphatic ducts.

Leukemia and its related diseases function in the same manner. A typical sign of leukemia is a large number of leukemic cells and a loss of their function as defensive cells (as well as a decrease of neutrophillic granulocytes). But since the bone marrow permits leukemic cells to enter into the bloodstream more quickly than do other organs, leukemia usually becomes quickly apparent in the blood and is easy to recognize. The organs in which leukemia develops are the location in which normal cells form until they turn into leukemic cells: bone marrow, lymph nodes, spleen. Like any other tumor cell, leukemic cells destroy the organ in which they originate, in this case bone marrow and lymph nodes.

▶ *Acute and Chronic Mycloid (Granulocytic) Leukemia and the Philadelphia Chromosome*

Mycloid leukemia develops from the precursor cells of the granulocytes. A characteristic feature of chronic myelocytic leukemia (CML) is an anomaly of the nuclei known as the Philadelphia chromosome which can be seen with special cytogenetic techniques under a microscope. Its presence confirms the diagnosis of chronic myelocytic leukemia.

Both acute myelocytic leukemia (AML) and CML are identified in the laboratory by the large number of leukocytes. As a rule the number of leukocytes increases to several tens of thousands times that of white blood corpuscles. Cell differentiation under the microscope will detect predominantly granulocytic cell types. As with other malignant tumors, these cells show signs of malignant changes. With AML this degeneration is more advanced than in cases of CML. These cells are also called immature cells (or blasts). As they degenerate there is a widespread loss of cell function.

▶ *Other Forms of Leukemia*

Nearly all the cells formed in our bone marrow can degenerate into forms of leukemia. Thus there is leukemia of the monocytes, of the preliminary forms of thrombocytes (the megakaryocytes), and of eosinophil leukocytes. Compared to the forms described previously, however, these are much more rare. Diagnosis always requires tests of both the blood and the bone marrow. The various forms of leukemia have different prognoses and treatments.

▶ *Blood Lab Tests for Chronic Leukemia and Acute Leukemia*

The blood picture is the first indicator in these cases because of the significantly increased number of leukocytes (30,000 to 50,000 per microliter). A differential blood count will help determine the affected cell type. If the leukocytes' nuclei contain a Philadelphia chromosome it is a case of CML. If the cells show signs of more severe degeneration and other changes studied with cytochemistry one can conclude that it is AML.

Testing of the bone marrow will be necessary for further differential diagnosis, and for assessment of the bone marrow's tumor involvement.

▶ *Cancer of the Lymphatic System*

Tumors of the lymphatic system constitute the largest portion of all blood cancers. They include a number of diseases with very different developments and symptoms.

Acute lymphatic leukemia (ALL), for example, is a common form of cancer in children. Chronic lymphatic leukemia (CLL), on the other hand, tends to occur more frequently in later life. In both the number of leukocytes in the blood picture is usually drastically increased. Cell counts often exceed 100,000 in a microliter of blood. Differential tests of the blood smear show that more than 90 percent of these cells are lymphocytes. Concurrent with the increase in the number of lymphocytes the lymph nodes grow until there is a noticeable, widespread lymph node swelling. For this reason the term lymph node cancer has become widely used.

Apart from these two types of lymphatic leukemia, there are other and more rare tumors of the lymphatic system. They are differentiated by complicated microscopic and lab chemical marker tests which use monoclonal antibodies to make certain structures within or on the surface of the leukemic cells visible. However, these tests can be performed only by highly specialized laboratories.

HODGKIN AND NON-HODGKIN LYMPHOMA   Two common forms of lymph node tumors should also be mentioned. Hodgkin's lymphoma was first described at the beginning of the 19th century by its discoverer, after which it is named. This disease produces typical cells that are visible in lymph node biopsies and are known as Reed-Sternberg cells. It occurs most frequently between the ages of 15 and 50 years. Changes in the blood picture are not characteristic and for a diagnosis it is necessary to surgically remove an enlarged lymph node.

The same diagnostic procedure is used for non-Hodgkin lymphomas. These do not produce the same changes in the cells and usually occur later in life. Neither type of tumor can be diagnosed on the basis of a blood picture alone.

SUMMARY

A diagnosis of leukemia can usually be suspected from the blood picture alone. In cases of chronic myelomonocytic leukemia (CML) a blood smear is sufficient to confirm the diagnosis. Chronic lymphatic leukemia is also sufficiently typical that a differential blood picture will confirm the diagnosis. To diagnose rare forms of leukemia and tumors of lymphatic origin, tissue samples of the bone marrow or of the affected lymph nodes have to be taken. An exact classification is often possible only by using special methods.

►► *AIDS—A Virus That Weakens the Body's Defenses*

AIDS (acquired immunodeficiency syndrome) is an infectious disease caused by a virus. The virus has been named after the disease which it causes: HIV[1] (human immunodeficiency virus). It belongs to a group of viruses which have been known to the medical profession for some time. HIV[1] (also known as HTLV III) attacks certain blood lymphocytes of the T4 type, brain cells, and intestinal cells. This pattern of involvement explains the symptoms that are caused by the disease which include infections, diarrhea, weight loss, mental and neurologic changes, and secondary cancers. Mortality is high. Despite the fact that tests in Africa have shown that HIV is not a new virus, the disease itself and its connection to HIV was discovered in the Western world only in the early 1980's. The impetus came from unexplained deaths among homosexuals in San Francisco.

To this day in the Western hemisphere the disease affects predominantly men. However, male and female drug addicts and patients infected with transfused blood or blood products (hemophiliacs) account for other victims of AIDS. Prevention must address changes in high-risk behavior. These include the use of condoms; use of clean, sterile needles; and control of blood products by meticulous screening.

The ratio of infected men and women in Africa is 1:1. Also in Africa significantly more children are infected than in America or Europe.

Despite the fact that there are infectious diseases in the world which affect and even kill much greater numbers of people, AIDS has had a greater impact on our consciousness. The mixture of social values and deadly disease has brought about a notoriety that has elevated AIDS to be considered the epidemic of the century.

▶ *AIDS Has Many Faces*

AIDS is an infectious disease. Its behavior is comparable to all other infectious diseases, and accordingly involves a number of different stages. In the beginning there is often an acute illness which appears to be a viral infection with uncharacteristic symptoms. Fever, joint pains, a frequently short-lived rash and temporary swelling of the lymph nodes will last only a few days or, rarely, weeks. Frequently, appearances suggest flu. In some cases there are no symptoms at all. After a latent period of months or even years, a painless swelling of the lymph nodes may occur. This stage is known as lymphadenopathic syndrome (LAS). It too may spontaneously disappear again, or transform into the stage of fullblown AIDS.

At this stage infections appear which are less common. They include opportunistic infections by fungi which attack the esophagus, and by germs (pneumocystis carinii) which attack the lungs. At this stage there will often be neurological symptoms. The appearance of a tumor which primarily affects the skin, the Kaposi-sarcoma, is typical for AIDS.

▶ High-Risk Groups

In North America and Europe, AIDS is not a disease like measles or chickenpox, that everyone is equally likely to contract. AIDS research has shown that some groups of people are significantly more at risk than the average population. This increased risk is because these people are more likely, over the course of their lifetime, to come into direct contact with the HIV. They are primarily homosexuals, intravenous drug users, hemophiliacs, as well as medical and nursing professionals. Particularly at risk are the children of HIV-infected mothers. This is how HIV is frequently transmitted in Africa, and is the reason why many African children are infected.

▶ Blood Lab Test for AIDS

Soon after the discovery of HIV, a test was developed for detecting the infection. The standard test can detect the presence of substances which our body forms to defend itself against the virus (HIV antibodies). But this test has a number of drawbacks. It can be used to demonstrate an infection only after 8 to 12 weeks have elapsed, and in various cases with a low likelihood of HIV infection it will falsely indicate the presence of antibodies, and therefore of HIV. That is why a positive test result alone is not considered sufficient to diagnose AIDS or one of the stages of HIV infection.

In the early stage of an infection only the virus itself can be detected in the blood, since the body will not yet have formed any antibodies. During this phase only specialized laboratories are equipped to detect components of the virus. For the specific detection of HIV antibodies, a special test, called the Western-blot-method is used. It, too, will show positive results only 12 weeks after the infection. It is used, however, to confirm an initial, positive HIV test. Only when the two tests are combined can one make any definitive statement about the presence of an HIV infection.

During the lymphadenopathic stage, and during fully manifested AIDS, typical changes in the blood picture will occur. The invasion of the virus lowers the amount of lymphocytes present in the blood. Typically the number of T4-lymphocytes will be reduced. These cells can be detected only by a special method of differentiating lympho-cytes which involves monoclonal antibodies, and which can be per-formed only by specially equipped laboratories.

These changes, however, are typical not only for AIDS. The num-ber of T4-lymphocytes will also decrease over the course of different viral infections and diseases of the immune system, which means that they cannot be used by themselves to diagnose AIDS. Only a combina-tion of clinical findings and lab tests can determine a diagnosis of AIDS.

SUMMARY

AIDS is an infectious disease. As with all infectious diseases it involves a series of stages. These can frequently last for years. Certain typical clinical pictures are known: lymphadeno-pathic syndrome (LAS) and fullblown AIDS, involving oppor-tunistic infections and Kaposi-sarcoma. Detection of the disease is based on laboratory-chemical detection of HIV anti-bodies. A diagnosis becomes probable only if two indepen-dent tests have shown positive results. If a patient belongs to a high-risk group, and if both tests show positive results, then a diagnosis of AIDS or its preliminary stages is so probable as to be almost a certainty. Lymphocyte differentiation can be used as a further diagnostic aid, but its results are not typical for AIDS alone.

5

THE HEART AND CARDIOVASCULAR SYSTEM

►► *The Heart's Central Role in the Circulatory System*

For human beings the heart has always played a central role. It is the uncontested symbol of love, and people whose heart is "in the right place" are considered honest and likeable. In medicine the heart also plays a central role. It is the motor in the infinitely branching network of large, small, and tiny blood vessels through which our blood continually flows.

The heart's development from the simple muscular tube (still found in many simple organisms) to a system with four chambers, takes place in every fetus in the womb. Disruptions during its maturation into a complex organ, such as viral infections during the first weeks of pregnancy, can cause congenital heart defects. In particular, infections with German measles during the first trimester of pregnancy have been known to cause malformations. In order to alleviate any fear of this danger, pregnant women are tested at the beginning of their pregnancy in order to determine if there is an immunity against German measles.

► *The Structure of Our Heart*

Over the course of our lives, the heart's weight increases until it reaches about nine and a half ounces (300 grams) in adults. Through

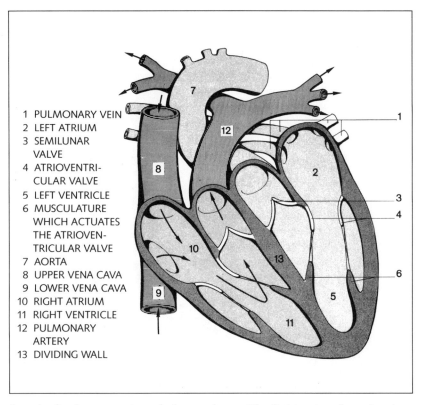

1 PULMONARY VEIN
2 LEFT ATRIUM
3 SEMILUNAR
   VALVE
4 ATRIOVENTRI-
   CULAR VALVE
5 LEFT VENTRICLE
6 MUSCULATURE
   WHICH ACTUATES
   THE ATRIOVEN-
   TRICULAR VALVE
7 AORTA
8 UPPER VENA CAVA
9 LOWER VENA CAVA
10 RIGHT ATRIUM
11 RIGHT VENTRICLE
12 PULMONARY
   ARTERY
13 DIVIDING WALL

Longitudinal cross section of a human heart. The division into four chambers is clearly visible.

exercise and sports, however, the heart can increase its weight significantly. We are familiar with this principle from our visible muscles which increase in bulk and size when we train in specific ways, as in body building. Since our heart's main mass consists of muscle tissue it is able to adapt to increased demands by increasing muscle mass. This amount of growth is limited, however, by the heart muscle's own blood supply system.

In us and in all mammals, the heart is situated at a functionally central location between the lungs and the body's circulation system. Anatomically, most of the heart is situated at the center of the chest cavity. The heart's tip (apex), which can be felt in the left side of the chest, marks the tip of the left heart chamber (ventricle). There are also a right ventricle and a left and right atrium. Blood flows from the right atrium through the right ventricle into the lung's circulatory system, and then through the left atrium (or auricle) into the left ven-

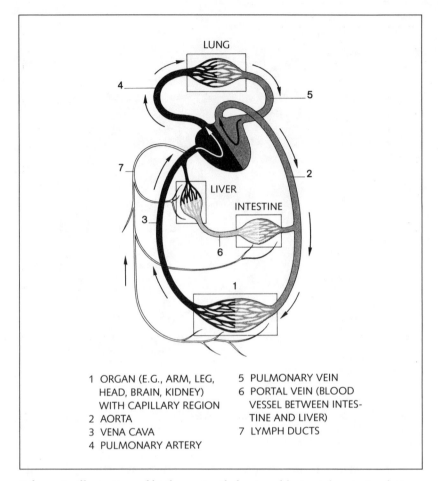

LUNG

4

5

7

2

LIVER

INTESTINE

3

6

1

1 ORGAN (E.G., ARM, LEG, HEAD, BRAIN, KIDNEY) WITH CAPILLARY REGION
2 AORTA
3 VENA CAVA
4 PULMONARY ARTERY

5 PULMONARY VEIN
6 PORTAL VEIN (BLOOD VESSEL BETWEEN INTES-TINE AND LIVER)
7 LYMPH DUCTS

Schematic illustration of both greater (below) and lesser (above) circulation

tricle, and from there through the aorta to the systemic circulation.

Auricles and ventricles are separated by valves. These allow the blood to flow only in one direction. At the openings towards the lungs and the body's circulation there are also valves in order to optimize the blood flow into these two systems. If we compare the heart valves to a car engine they are the equivalent of the combustion chamber's intake and exhaust valves.

► *Structure and Function of Our Circulation System*

THE STRUCTURE OF OUR CIRCULATION   Our circulation is schematically divided into the greater (or systemic) and the lesser (or pulmonary) circulation. The terms greater and lesser refer to the total areas of the two circulations, each of which covers several square yards. These large areas are needed for our metabolism. The right ventricle, the lung's blood vessels, and the left atrium (or auricle) taken together are called the lesser (pulmonary) circulation. The greater (systemic) circulation consists of the left ventricle, the body's circulation system and the right atrium.

SUMMARY

Our heart and circulation are one system. The heart is a large muscle which has been transformed over the course of our evolutionary development into a system of four enclosed chambers through which the blood is transported. By actively contracting the chambers our heart propels the blood through the greater and lesser circulations.

HOW OUR CIRCULATION WORKS   Our greater and lesser circulations function like the water supply and sewer system of a large city. Pipelines are used to pump fresh water into the houses where it is used for cooking, washing, and cleaning. Waste water flows through the drainpipes into sewage treatment plants where the impurities are filtered out, and the water is returned into the fresh water cycle.

In our circulation system this means that oxygen-rich blood from the lung's circulation is pumped into the body circulation by the left ventricle. The blood then supplies various organs, collects their waste products, and finally returns to collect in the large veins and to flow back to the right heart. From there it is pumped into the lung circulation where gaseous waste products are released with the breath, and the blood is charged with fresh oxygen to start a new cycle.

To maintain a constant flow of blood, our heart beats more than 100,000 times a day, and more than 25 million times during the seventy-five years of our life. The total amount of blood that has to be moved in a day is more than 1,700 gallons (7,000 liters). And there is no time for repairs!

OUR VASCULAR SYSTEM   Using our example of the automobile, one can compare our blood vessels to the various roads of our traffic system. If we did not have highways, city roads, and alleys we would not be able to get to our homes and workplaces in an orderly way. Streets are to a traffic system what both arteries and veins are to our circulation system. For example, the blood vessels that we see on our hands and legs are veins.

HIGH AND LOW PRESSURE   This is how we distinguish between the arterial and the venous part of our circulation system. When the left ventricle contracts in order to pump blood into the body, it generates high pressure. The highest point of this pressure curve is called systolic pressure. The lowest point of the pressure curve in the arterial blood vessels is called the diastolic pressure. Normal systolic blood pressure values are between 100 and 140 mmHg (pressure in millimeters of mercury). This is the pressure with which the blood is first pumped from the left ventricle into the large artery (aorta). Because of the high pressure, arteries have thicker walls than veins. Areas that are subject to high pressure and have blood vessels constructed like arteries are called high pressure areas or arterial areas. As a rule, arterial areas contain oxygenated blood—with one exception: the area where blood flows in from the right ventricle through the lung's artery and into the lungs. This is where blood filled with certain waste products is pumped into the lung circulation.

The low pressure region is called the venous system. Since they have to withstand less pressure, these blood vessels, the veins, have thinner walls. The largest vein in our body is the upper and lower vena cava (from the Latin *cavus:* hollow), which conducts blood back to the heart. Because they are flexible, veins can act like a blood reservoir. This quality can be used to help someone who has fainted by raising their legs to stabilize their blood pressure, which helps them regain consciousness.

▶ *The Metabolism in Our Capillaries*

The many branchings of our arteries whose diameter diminishes from two inches (5 centimeters) in the aorta to only thousandths of a millimeter in the capillaries, helps to lower the pressure in the blood vessels. These extremely fine blood vessels, which all together are called the capillary bed, are where the actual exchange of substances (metabolism) in our organs takes place. This region is the watershed between the high pressure and low pressure systems of our body.

▸▸ *Cardiac Arrest—Killer Number One*

▸ *Acute and Chronic Heart Failure*

If our heart stops, we die. If this happens, as is increasingly common, in an intensive care unit one can observe on a monitor how the heart's electric impulses grow weaker and weaker. This state is frequently the result of a more or less lengthy development, but its conclusion is a complete failure of the heart.

In some cases, heart failure occurs suddenly, as sudden cardiac arrest. Its causes are often impossible to determine after the fact. These deaths have no previous symptoms. Since symptoms can often mean long periods of suffering before death, there are people who wish for a sudden cardiac arrest, saying that they simply want to be struck dead without warning. The opposite phenomenon is the heart sufferer who spends a long time suffering from symptoms caused by the diseased heart. In both cases the heart fails and the circulation stops. How does this happen?

THE CAUSES OF HEART FAILURE   The heart is a powerful muscle that encloses a number of hollow chambers. When the heart muscle contracts, it pumps blood into the circulation. This pumping action keeps the circulation running. Coordination and control of the pumping performance is provided by the heart's electrical system, which is responsible for our heart's rhythm.

Heart failure can be caused either by the electrical system or by the muscular pumping system. Sudden death in heart attacks is usually due to a disruption of the electrical system. Since these rhythmic disruptions can be treated relatively easily during a heart attack's inital stages, early efforts at reviving the patient are often successful.

HEART FAILURE DUE TO TOTAL OCCLUSION   Our heart is equipped with several electrical systems. One of them conducts electricity from the anterior chamber (atrium) towards the ventricles, while another helps spread the impulses throughout the ventricles. If the anterior system is disrupted, impulses cannot reach the ventricles, and the heart may stop pumping. This is known as a total block between auricle and ventricle (an A-V block). If conductivity is disrupted in the main chambers we speak of an interventricular (or bundle branch) heart block. Given the large muscle mass of the heart chamber, a blockage forces the electric impulses to travel far, and an interventricular electrical blockage is the result. The EKG (electrocardiogram) records the normal electrical impulses in the heart in the

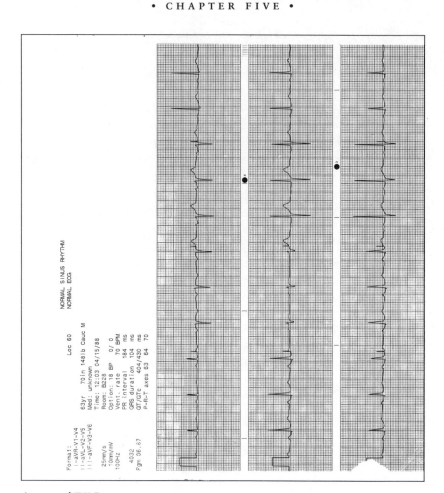

A normal EKG

form of an EKG-curve. Disruptions of the impulse path, as in a block-age, lead to characteristic electrical current patterns, which are known as an EKG-picture of an interventricular blockage.

Depending on which chamber is primarily affected, it is known as either a left or a right interventricular blockage. A short circuit may result, causing a chaotic series of electric signals in the areas where the impulse is formed and conducted, and as a result pumping action becomes ineffective or ceases. The picture seen on a heart monitor, for example is one of fibrillation (irregular spasms). Once this happens everything suddenly stops, and we are confronted with a sudden cardiovascular arrest.

HOW THE EKG (ELECTROCARDIOGRAM) WORKS   As these cardiac

disruptions are invisible to the naked eye, it is often difficult to determine the cause of sudden cardiac death, unless, of course, an electrocardiogram was being made at the time.

The EKG helps to make the heart's conduction system visible. By applying metallic electrodes to the wrists, ankles, and chest, the heart's currents can be detected and graphically recorded. The shape, frequency, distances between, and duration of the recorded impulses provide insights into the ordered and disordered electrical processes inside the heart. If the EKG shows a series of extra heartbeats in between the beats of the normal (sinus) rhythm, this indicates arrhythmia (from the Greek *arrhuthmos:* without rhythm). Most people have experienced this merely as a "stumbling" or momentary stopping of the heartbeat. For a person suffering from heart disease, however, these variations can have serious or even fatal consequences. For this reason the EKG by itself can only rarely indicate whether someone has a healthy heart or not. One reason is that the EKG records only electrical phenomena without providing information about the strength of the heart muscle and its pumping function.

▶ *Heart Insufficiency*

When someone is suffering from gradually progressive heart failure this becomes visible even to a lay person. In these cases one can recognize the disease by changes in the person's body as symptoms become evident.

This complex of complaints is known as a heart insufficiency. The term expresses the heart's insufficient ability to supply the body with the necessary blood flow. At first the insufficiency becomes noticeable only during physical exertion, as when someone is unable to climb stairs because they feel short of breath. Towards the end a stage is reached where any but the the smallest movements create an intolerable feeling of asphyxiation.

If the right heart is no longer able to transport blood from the large circulation into the lungs, then the blood becomes congested in the large veins. The veins of the neck protrude, and sitting or standing for extended periods leads to a swelling of the legs, called edema. This condition is easy to recognize because the legs feel like liquid-filled cushions. Pressing a finger on the skin of the tibia leaves a pitting or a dimple for some time afterwards. As soon as the patients lie down, however, the blood can flow back more easily to the heart and the edema disappears again. Patients often report in these cases that every morning their legs have grown slim again. These symptoms indicate a disruption of the heart's function. They don't reveal the causes, however. If the left side of the heart fails, the lungs become congested and the patient is short of breath (dyspneic).

The diseases which most commonly lead to heart failure are:
• arteriosclerosis
• coronary heart disease (occlusion of the coronary blood vessels)
• increased arterial blood pressure (hypertension)
• congenital or acquired heart valve defects
• diseases of the heart muscle (cardiomyopathy)

The first three diseases are the "killers" of our society. Nearly every second man and every third woman dies from the consequences of one of these three diseases, which is why we called cardiac disease killer number one.

CHOLESTEROL AND ARTERIOSCLEROSIS   The original causes of arteriosclerosis, of coronary disease, and of hypertension can be completely different. However, they all cause damage to the blood vessels of our arterial circulation.

In the arterial walls more and more cholesterol, a blood lipid (fat) is deposited. This leads to the formation of cholesterol patches which break up, and, by injuring the arterial walls, trigger further thrombotic deposits. The result is that the arteries' clear diameter (lumen) becomes progressively smaller—up to total occlusion. The result is a decrease in blood flow leading to an insufficient supply of blood and nutrients to our organs. The visible signs of such an occlusion are a heart attack, a stroke, and leg ulcers.

Research has shown that this process can be speeded up or slowed down, depending on the amount of blood cholesterol and other lipids, and that cholesterol and these lipids are therefore an important, measurable indicator of arteriosclerosis.

ACQUIRED AND CONGENITAL FAT METABOLISM DISORDERS These cardiac disruptions are not always related to a person's diet. We know of some congenital fat metabolism disorders which cause even children to suffer from arteriosclerotic occlusions in their blood vessels. These children often die at an early age, and from causes such as heart attacks.

More frequent, however, are acquired fat metabolism disorders that are caused by an increased supply of dietary fats. Developments after the second World War have shown that dietary choices and eating habits have a direct influence. Our diet and its components have changed with our growing affluence, and proportions of both calories

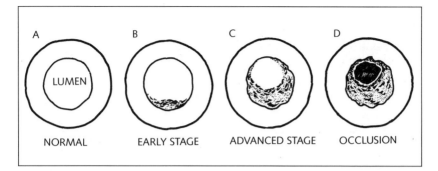

Development of arteriosclerosis in a normal artery (a), leading to complete occlusion (d)

and of fat in our food have increased. To what extent a progressive lack of roughage in our diet also contributes to an increased risk of arteriosclerosis still remains an open question.

▶ Blood Lab Test for Blood Lipids

Blood testing for lipids can be a valuable source of information. The most important component of blood fat testing is to determine the cholesterol level. Values of no more than 200 mg/dl are desirable; a slight increase may be acceptable later in life. It is important to determine levels for both HDL-cholesterol (the "good" cholesterol) and LDL-cholesterol (the "bad" cholesterol). The ratio between the two cholesterol subgroups helps us better estimate the risk of arteriosclerotic disease. In general, we can say the higher the proportion of HDL-cholesterol and the lower the LDL-cholesterol the lower will be the risk of arteriosclerosis.

BLOOD FATS

Cholesterol
HDL-cholesterol
LDL-cholesterol
triglyceride

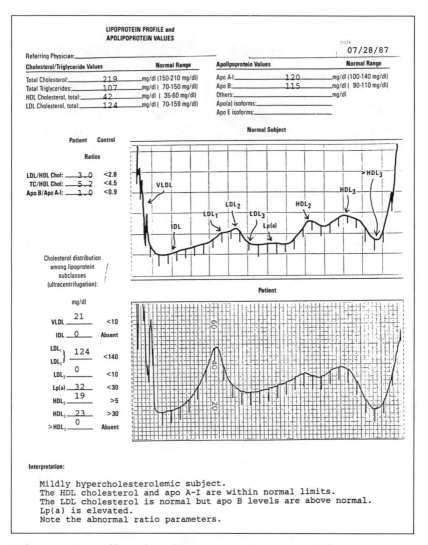

A lipoprotein profile and apolipoprotein values; normal/abnormal patient report

Important note: If you have elevated blood fat levels, or if several members of your family have suffered early in life either from arteriosclerosis or from coronary heart disease, you should start having your own blood fat levels monitored early in life. But blood fat levels are not the only factor in developing arteriosclerosis and coronary heart disease. It is important to note that smoking, high blood pressure, being overweight, and using oral contraceptives also increase the risk.

We know that athletic exercise or endurance training do not necessarily decrease the total cholesterol level, but they do shift the balance in favor of the good (HDL) cholesterol. Fish oil, which consists mainly of unsaturated fatty acids, has been found to be useful in increasing HDL-cholesterol levels. (Medical records of Greenland eskimos who hardly ever suffer from coronary heart disease, or arteriosclerosis, provided the original impulse to research these relationships.)

▶▶ *Early Detection of a Cardiac Infarct*

In the U.S.A. alone, over 1.5 million people have cardiac infarcts a year, and 35 percent die from such a heart attack. An additional 15 to 20 percent of victims die within the first year. (In Canada, each year there are about 175,000 heart attacks in a population of twenty-six million.) Heart attacks are the most common cause of death for men in North America. Alarming statistics show that the average age for infarct patients is decreasing to the forties.

We know that the most dangerous phase of an infarct is near the onset. Almost half of all fatalities due to heart attacks occur within the first four hours after the infarct has appeared. Sudden death usually occurs following disruptions of the heart's rhythm. Recent scientific studies have shown that the effectiveness of medical countermeasures is greatest during the early phase of the infarct.

These results prove what we have always suspected about heart attacks: the sooner something is done the better. How can we explain this danger? And how can it be minimized?

▶ *Angina Pectoris: The Warning Signs*

An important early warning system against the threat of a heart attack—one which is independent of age—is familiarity with one's risk factors. High blood fat values, smoking, a genetic predisposition, and high blood pressure are among the most important ones.

Angina pectoris, a feeling of constriction in the chest cavity, is a very precise warning signal for an impending heart attack. Once more than 50 percent of the blood vessel's diameter is constricted, the likelihood that these symptoms will develop increases steadily. The symptoms always appear when the relationship between oxygen supply and demand in the heart muscle is no longer properly balanced. When the two become disproportionate, this triggers the angina pectoris.

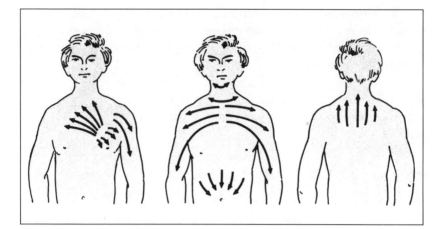

Localization and radiation of chest pain with angina pectoris

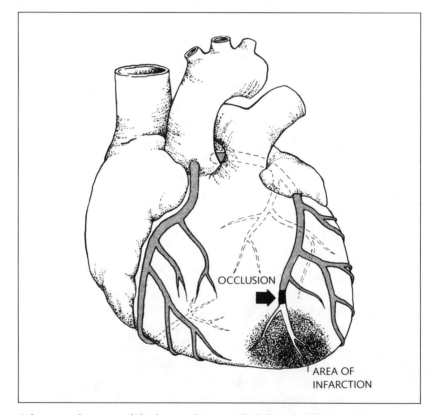

OCCLUSION

AREA OF
INFARCTION

*Schematic diagram of the heart, showing the left and right coronary arteries.
An infarction has occurred in the region of the heart's tip (apex), due to an
occlusion of the left branch of the coronary artery.*

The sensation of constriction is not the only symptom of angina pectoris, which, in fact, encompasses an entire complex of symptoms. Some of the more important individual symptoms will be briefly mentioned here. Bear in mind, however, that it is always your physician, and not you yourself, who should make the diagnosis. For this reason you should see your physician as soon as symptoms appear.

• Type of pain: This can differ widely. The spectrum ranges from pressure behind the sternum, "stitches" in the rib cage, a sensation of heaviness, and up to intensive crippling pain causing mortal fear in the patient. Patients commonly feel that their rib cage is being compressed as if by a vise.

• Localization of the pain: Typically, pain appears in the left half of the chest. Normally there is no definite point of origin that can be pinpointed. In some cases, for example, if the heart's posterior wall is suffering from a lack of oxygen, the pain can also be localized in the pit of the stomach.

• Radiation of pain: In some cases an actual chest pain is not perceived, but rather its radiation. Thus patients report pain in their left arm, mostly on the underside, and reaching all the way down to the fingers. Or it may be that the left mandibular joint (the joint of the lower jaw) is suddenly painful. Often massage therapy is erroneously prescribed to alleviate shoulder pains which actually stem from the heart.

• The trigger for an attack: Physical exertion leads to an increased oxygen demand which a diseased coronary system cannot fulfill. Increased psychological stress, extreme differences in temperature, and heavy meals can also trigger an attack of angina pectoris. In light attacks the pain disappears quickly once the physical stress has stopped. However, the fear of triggering an attack can lead to severe psychological disruptions. For example, in men this can cause a loss of libido and even impotence.

• The nitroglycerin test: Nitroglycerin taken as a sublingual tablet (under the tongue), causes arteries to dilate and heart muscle tone to decrease. These changes diminish the oxygen requirement of the heart muscle. If the requirements decrease until they are met even with constricted coronary arteries, the pain will disappear. If the pain is localized in the heart muscle and its blood vessels, this will happen in a few minutes. For this reason the nitroglycerin test is a diagnostic tool. After biting on a capsule or two inhalations of a nitroglycerin spray the patient soon feels an improvement.

If all five of these typical criteria are being fulfilled we speak of a typical angina. As a rule, this also means a diagnosis of coronary heart disease. It is often unnecessary to conduct other and more complicated tests. But just as often the situation is less unequivocal. Other diseases in neighboring organs can mimic the pain of an angina pectoris attack. For example, pain coming from the esophagus, the stomach, the pancreas, or the spine can appear like a symptom of coronary heart disease.

The most precise method of detecting coronary heart disease is the examination by cardiac catheter. For this, the patient is usually transferred to a special department. There a catheter is introduced into the groin or the elbow and slid forward until it reaches the heart. Special catheters are used to inject contrast media (substances which are opaque to x-rays) into the coronary arteries, making them visible on x-ray film. The specialist can then determine the extent and precise location of the occlusion. At the same time, it is now possible to introduce special instruments through the catheter which are used to widen the coronary stenosis, i.e. the narrowing in the artery, and so prevent an infarction. This process is known as angioplasty.

UNSTABLE AND STABLE ANGINA PECTORIS Many people know that they suffer from angina pectoris. They have learned to live with it, because they know under what circumstances they will suffer pain from an attack. This state is called stable angina pectoris. As long as this state is kept unchanged with the help of medication or surgery, the risk factor it poses is relatively low. However, if the pain increases in severity with little exertion, or if the type or intensity of the pain changes, or if attacks last longer, these are warning signals of an impending heart attack. Under these conditions we speak of an unstable angina pectoris. Because of the increased risk of suffering a heart attack from a state of unstable angina pectoris, it is also known as pre-infarction syndrome. In such a situation a physician must be called immediately, and it is urgent that the patient seeks admission to a hospital equipped with a coronary care unit. Here medication can be used to counteract the imminent heart attack at an early stage.

HOW THE EKG IS USED IN HEART ATTACKS In most cases with definite symptoms the EKG is the best way to determine whether an infarct has already occurred or not. We often find that in the early stages before an infarct, EKG wave amplitudes are shallower, while an actual infarct in the same place results in larger EKG wave amplitudes. Your physician is qualified to interpret these. That is why it is advisable to visit a physician early to have one's EKG explained.

In many cases, only a comparison with an earlier EKG can lead to a final diagnosis. This is why patients who already know that they have a coronary disease should carry their last EKG with them, to make comparisons possible in an emergency.

▶ *Blood Lab Test for Cardiac Infarct*

In this situation blood tests help the physician confirm the suspicion of a cardiac infarct. Three laboratory tests can indicate an infarct: Determining values of creatinekinase (CK), especially the muscle-specific types of CK (CK–MB), GOT, and LDH. Laboratory results are expressed in U/l (units per liter). CK can reach values of more than 1,000 units. These laboratory values show a typical sequence over time. CK appears first, followed by GOT and LDH. As a rule, laboratory values return to a completely normal level ten to fourteen days after an infarct without complications.

LAB TEST FOR CARDIAC INFARCTS

Creatinekinase (CK)
Glutamate-oxalate-transaminase (GOT)
Lactate dehydrogenase (LDH)

Important notes: During extreme physical exertion, muscle inflammation (myositis), and during brain infarcts, CK values can be elevated although there is no cardiac infarct. An assessment of clinical symptoms, of risk factors, and of the findings from a detailed examination, particularly from the EKG (electrocardiogram) can be helpful in correcting the diagnosis. This is why a laboratory test must always be viewed in combination with the clinical findings.

Two methods can provide information about the extent of an infarct. There is a direct correlation between the maximum measured CK values and the size of the heart muscle region that has died. The EKG also allows an estimate of the infarct's extent.

SUMMARY

Arteriosclerosis of the coronary arteries leads to coronary heart disease. It appears in a variety of stages which can blend with one another. The most severe and life-threatening form is the cardiac infarct. If it announces itself by early symptoms, prompt countermeasures by the physician can prevent serious consequences. Important examinations in this context include the electrocardiogram, laboratory testing for certain enzymes, medication, heart catheterization, and most importantly the patient's cooperation.

▶▶ *Prevention is Better than Treatment*

In the future, physicians will be more and more concerned with problems of prevention. Even though the rate of fatalities among heart attack patients has decreased due to modern medical methods there will always be a certain percentage of deaths. As a result of its characteristics, and of the heart's central role in our organism, cardiac disease always involves a mortal risk. In order to lower the fatality rate, specific efforts are necessary to eliminate those factors that lead to cardiac infarcts and coronary heart disease.

▶ *Risk Factors*

At this time there is consensus that high blood pressure, fat metabolism disorders, diabetes mellitus, smoking, excessive weight, and lack of exercise are all risk factors. And one must keep in mind that combinations of two or more of these factors increase the risk of sickness exponentially. It is possible that genetic factors play an additional role in favoring the development of coronary heart disease. Probably these genetic factors are the hidden causes behind special diseases, such as diseases of the blood vessels, whose significance is not yet understood. All these factors taken together are called the "coronary risk." Every single person has an individual coronary risk, and the sum of the individual factors we have mentioned result in your personal coronary risk. After reading the following section you will be able to draw up your own coronary risk profile.

RISK FACTOR: BLOOD PRESSURE (HYPERTENSION) We distinguish between two different forms of high blood pressure. Whenever medical science cannot explain a phenomenon it uses the convention of calling the phenomenon "essential," or "idiopathic" (from the Greek *idios:* separate, and *pathos:* suffering, thus "a disease having its own origin"). Thus, we refer to the form of hypertension whose cause is not clearly understood as "essential hypertension."

By contrast, there are forms of hypertension which can be traced back to diseases in other organs which eventually lead to hypertension. Among these we count diseases of the hormone glands, of the kidneys' arteries, of the large body artery (aortic stenosis), and of the heart valves (aortic insufficiency). These all lead to what we call secondary hypertension. This condition is rare and constitutes only about five percent of the total number of cases of hypertension. The damage which the two forms cause is the same, however. To determine the risk requires only a simple procedure: regular blood pressure measurement by your family doctor.

Among the general population certain groups are more at risk of developing hypertension than others. For children of hypertensive mothers there is a significant risk. These children often have elevated blood pressure at an early age.

Normal blood pressure values are up to 140 mmHg for the systolic value and 90 mmHg for the diastolic value. If one of the two values is exceeded at rest—up to 150 mmHg systolic and over 90 mmHg diastolic—this means that the value has reached a grey area and frequent monitoring will be needed.

It is not enough to measure blood pressure only once, because it will vary with the time of day, and is also affected by the degree of physical and mental stress during measurement. This is why measurements taken at the physician's office tend to be higher than measurements taken at home. Thus it is only sensible to try to be as relaxed as possible when blood pressure is being measured, and not to do it immediately after physical exertion.

In young people who have increased blood pressure in their arms one must definitely also measure pressure in the legs. Then, if blood pressure is normal in the legs, it may be a case of aortic stenosis which belongs to the group of secondary hypertension, which can be corrected surgically.

RISK FACTOR: FAT METABOLISM DISORDERS Elevated cholesterol levels, in particular an increase in bad cholesterol (LDL) along with a decrease in good cholesterol (HDL) promotes the development of coronary heart disease and the formation of a cardiac infarct. If a genetic predisposition has been established for your family, it is very important that your blood fat values are monitored. This test is harmless for you, and will provide important information about your coronary risk.

The importance of this has been demonstrated by so-called

intervention-studies in which diet and/or medication were used to keep the cholesterol level and particularly the LDL-cholesterol level lower in one test group of people than in a control group. The group that was being treated suffered significantly fewer cardiac infarctions—proof that your blood fat value is a factor in your health.

RISK FACTOR: DIABETES MELLITUS Diabetes is discussed in detail in chapter 9. Here it will suffice to say that diabetes is a risk factor. By testing urine and blood it can be easily determined if diabetes is present or if there is a metabolic condition which promotes the development of diabetes.

RISK FACTOR: WEIGHT Once you have gone beyond your normal weight every pound increases your coronary risk. In most cases a metabolic disorder, or diabetes mellitus, also appears in connection with the weight. As these risk factors usually appear in combination it has not been researched in detail how much weight alone contributes to coronary risk.

RISK FACTOR: SMOKING In North America the rate of heart attacks has been declining for some years, and at the same time nicotine consumption has decreased. This is the best proof that by avoiding nicotine we can save lives. Not only does it save money but it is an investment in our future. Talk to your family doctor about the consequences of smoking. You will also lower your risk of developing lung cancer.

RISK FACTOR: LACK OF EXERCISE When you move your body you give your heart a workout. This work stresses the cardiovascular system. If you administer the exercise in well-proportioned doses you can train your heart to increase its oxygen supply when it has to work harder. To achieve this, the heart can increase its own coronary circulation and gradually adapt to the increased stress. It increases its coronary reserves. This coronary reserve in turn increases the ability of your heart to withstand stress, and brings about an increased efficiency of heart function. At the same time, fat metabolism is improved.

Endurance training teaches our body to use fat rather than sugar as the basis of energy conversion. The cholesterol level decreases, HDL-cholesterol increases, and coronary risk diminishes. But do not try to train yourself in a short time to be a marathon runner for one event only. Short term exertion and extreme stress have no effect on coronary risk.

You can see how much you yourself can do for your health. The idea that prevention is better than treatment has become popular with health insurance plans, as well, and many of them will cover the cost of an annual check-up. Talk to your physician about your health and about ways of maintaining it. Better safe than sorry.

6

LIVER AND GALL BLADDER

The development of our liver and gall bladder are closely connected during our maturation process. Our liver's function and structure are directly linked to the anatomical structure of the bile ducts, and the bile which flows in them. Among the products of our liver, bile is the most visible. This connection is even reflected in some of our common expressions, such as a "liverish" person is one whose "bile rises easily."

▶▶ *The Liver's Functions*

The liver is the largest organ in our body. Weighing about 3 pounds (1.5 kg), it is the largest single organ mass in our body after the musculature.

Its two primary functions can be described as removing poisonous substances (detoxification), and synthesizing a variety of compounds. These functions are like those of a chemical factory, where basic components are combined to form useful end products.

▶ *Detoxification*

As our detoxification organ the liver functions like a sewage treatment plant. In order to do this, however, it consumes a considerable amount of energy. Poisonous substances that have entered our body, whether they are medications, dietary poisons, or even poisonous stimulants, like alcohol, are broken down in the liver, and usually released as substances that are harmless to our organism. This remarkable performance is accomplished with the many different enzymes that equip our liver.

LIVER ENZYMES

Glutamate-pyruvate-transaminase (SGPT)
Glutamate-oxalacetate-transaminase (SGOT)
Alkaline phosphatase (AP or ALK.phos)
Cholinesterase (CHE)
Gamma-glutamyl-transferase (GGT)
Lactate dehydrogenase (LDH)

Our liver is like a filter built into our intestinal venous drainage system (portal vein). In the portal vein all the substances that have been absorbed from the intestine are transported to the liver. The liver's interior structure is like an extremely fine system of canals that are bordered by liver cells as the smallest functional units. Blood enters this system from the intestine's portal vein system, and the exit opens into the body's venous region and the large vena cava.

Our bile ducts begin as tiny bile capillaries in the liver and merge outside the liver into the cystic duct. They form a secondary canal system that is separated from the blood by the liver cells. These ducts collect the bile which our liver produces and which we need to digest food.

▶ *Synthetic Functions*

Because of its anatomical structure the liver is an important component in our food processing cycle. Since the basic substances of our diet are carbohydrates, proteins, and fats, our liver plays a central role in their metabolism.

The liver is our largest glycogen (carbohydrate) storage area—the region that synthesizes very important proteins and sees to it that the fats in our blood are bound to transport substances. This is done to prevent the fats from forming deposits in our blood vessels.

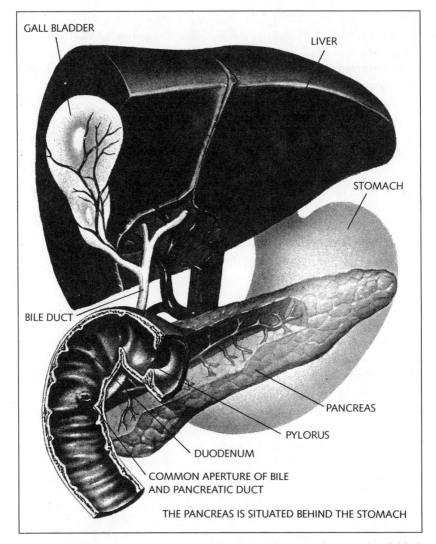

GALL BLADDER

LIVER

STOMACH

BILE DUCT

PANCREAS

PYLORUS

DUODENUM

COMMON APERTURE OF BILE
AND PANCREATIC DUCT

THE PANCREAS IS SITUATED BEHIND THE STOMACH

Schematic illustration showing the relationship between liver and gall blad-der, as well as bile ducts and duodenum. The position of stomach and pan-creas are also shown.

Bile production is another task for which our liver is exclusively responsible. The bile, of which about 3 quarts (1.5 liters) are pro-duced every day, is an important factor in our digestion, and provides another option for removing poisonous substances from the body. The bile's composition determines almost exclusively whether gall-stones will be formed. (See *The Gall Bladder*, p. 114.)

▶ *Blood Lab Test for Liver Function*

Because of its central role, any changes in liver function will always be reflected in our blood. If the liver cannot fulfill its task as our metabolic organ, the blood levels of carbohydrates (glucose), proteins (albumin), and fats (cholesterol) will change. Another central function of our liver is the production (synthesis) of important substances, like glycogen, clotting agents, and the proteins—the building blocks of our body.

If the liver's detoxification function comes to a halt, toxic substances collect in the blood, which can lead to symptoms of poisoning. If liver cells are damaged, their enzymes will be released into the blood and will exceed normal levels. If the liver cells are no longer able to produce bile, or if they can no longer release the bile into the bile ducts, the result will be a release of bile pigments into the blood, and eventually jaundice (icterus). (See page 118.)

In connection with this, our blood is especially useful in revealing our liver's functioning and its diseases.

▶▶ *You Don't Feel A Liver Disease*

Our liver has great regenerative powers. Even if half of the liver's tissue is removed, its function can be maintained fully, by means of regenerative processes. Thus it is not surprising that liver diseases produce few and often non-specific symptoms. For example, many people have already suffered from an inflammation of the liver (hepatitis) without knowing it. This was discovered once we had the means to detect the infection in the blood. It was also found that the rate of infection is particularly high in countries where hygienic conditions are poor.

▶ *Inflammation of the Liver (Hepatitis)*

The most common infectious disease of the liver is hepatitis. It is caused by a virus. An acute liver infection, which as a rule subsides after a few days or weeks, usually to be completely healed, is known as acute hepatitis. Its opposite is chronic hepatitis, which can turn into acute hepatitis. Chronic hepatitis is distinguished by the fact that liver enzyme values remain elevated six months after the initial infection.

The hepatitis viruses belong to a common group, but they differ from one another, so that, depending on the type of virus, we distinguish between hepatitis A (virus A), hepatitis B (virus B), hepatitis C (virus C), and in rare cases hepatitis D (virus D).

Before the various viruses were identified, hepatitis was classified according to its clinical development. Hepatitis A was called infectious hepatitis, since this form often appeared like an epidemic. Hepatitis B was called serum hepatitis, because its appearance had been observed following serum and blood transfusions.

One form which could be classified as neither hepatitis A nor hepatitis B was called hepatitis non-A-non-B. Since 1990 we have known that this form is caused by a virus, now called virus C.

Laboratory medicine has made a large contribution to understanding the viruses that cause these forms of hepatitis. Nowadays a serological test can be used to detect the infection. Blood examinations can also help distinguish between fresh infections and those that have already run their course.

HEPATITIS A (INFECTIOUS HEPATITIS) Since an infection with hepatitis A can come about through the consumption of food, the virus can be detected in the stool just a few days after the infection, and before any other changes in laboratory test results have appeared. During the struggle between the body's immune defense systems and the intruding virus, certain defensive substances known as antibodies (anti-HAV) are formed, and these can be detected in the blood after only a few weeks. In fresh or renewed infections with the hepatitis virus A (HAV), antibodies of the M class are formed. These can be distinguished in the blood from the G-class antibodies that are present if there is an immunity against HAV.

HEPATITIS B (SERUM HEPATITIS) The virus responsible for hepatitis B (HBV) can be detected mainly in the blood. At the earliest of one to two weeks after the infection, a test based on a reaction to certain parts of this virus (HBSAG) becomes positive. The virus intrudes in the liver cells and is transformed in such a way that the complete virus is no longer present in the bloodstream. But some detectable substances from the virus appear in the blood which can be identified by our immune system. They allow us to determine whether an infection is fresh or old and whether it is a still active or infectious form.

If HBSAG (hepatitis-B-surface-antigen) and e–AG (envelope antigen) are found in the blood, there is a danger of infection. If antibodies against these antigens are present (anti-HBs and anti-HBe) in connection with anti-HBc (antibodies against core-B-antigen), the disease has run its course, and there is no more danger of infection. The appearance of these blood components has been found regularly and is considered typical for many diseases. This is why the antigens and antibodies against hepatitis B virus are called "markers," indicating the development of the disease.

HEPATITIS B MARKERS

Hepatitis-B-surface-antigen (HBSAG)
Anti-hepatitis-B-surface (Anti-HBs)
Hepatitis-e-antigen (HBe-Ag)
Anti-hepatitis-e (Anti-HBe)
Anti-hepatitis-c (Anti-HBc)
Anti-hepatitis-c-IgM (Anti-HBc-IgM)

HEPATITIS C (NON-A-NON-B-HEPATITIS) At this time the only detection method for hepatitis C is the antibody detection of a part of the hepatitis C virus (HCV), which often takes twelve weeks after the infection to become positive. This form of liver infection is often caused by contaminated blood transfusions. Today it is known that in industrialized countries this form is the most common cause of chronic hepatitis.

In some countries, such as India, for example, infections can also occur through food. A serological test for HCV antibodies will be positive in these cases. Recent studies give us reason to suspect, however, that although these antibodies are identical, they are in fact being produced against another, related virus. It has been proposed to name this virus "E," and the inflammation it causes "hepatitis E."

HEPATITIS D (DELTA-HEPATITIS) In connection with hepatitis B infections, what we call a superinfection with a further part of the virus can occur. This form appears mainly in Mediterranean countries. For purposes of virus identification this form has been named "hepatitis D."

▶ *Blood Lab Test for Hepatitis*

As we have mentioned, liver cells are rich in enzymes. Typical liver enzymes, are alanine aminotransferase (ALT, SGPT) and aspartate aminotransferase (AST, SGOT), although these do not appear exclusively in the liver. Other important liver test values are gamma-glutamyl-transferase (GGT, gamma-GT), and alkaline phosphatase (AP). SGPT and SGOT are together known as transaminases. Their normal values are listed in the appendix of significant blood values.

LIVER ENZYMES PRESENT DURING HEPATITIS

Alanine aminotransferase (ALT, GPT, SGPT)
Aspartate aminotransferase (AST, SGOT)
Gamma-glutamyl-transferase (GGT, gamma-GT)
Alkaline phosphatase (AP)

If a virus leads to liver inflammation, liver cells die. The enzymes they contain are released and can be detected in the blood in increasing amounts. In connection with a liver infection, blood levels of SGPT and SGOT rise in a typical pattern. Measured values can reach several hundred units, in severe cases more than a thousand units. As a rule, SGPT values rise only slightly higher than SGOT values. Generally GGT and AP levels also rise. These laboratory values are sufficient to diagnose hepatitis with a high degree of probability, augmented by serological testing to classify the type of virus.

In connection with an increase in liver enzymes, often the only symptoms that appear are reminiscent of a flu. This is why in the presence of such symptoms the physician often orders enzyme values to be checked in the lab to determine whether the complaints are caused by hepatitis. These elevated measurements only last a few days and then slowly decrease to normal levels. This decrease can be used to monitor the process of recovery.

An unfavorable development is being signalled if transaminase levels drop very quickly to normal or below normal. This situation often indicates a massive incident of liver cell death that can lead to liver failure. Suddenly all liver functions cease. The result is a drop in glucose levels, bile production stops entirely, and the liver's synthesizing performance as measured by the blood levels of albumin comes to a halt. This acutely threatening clinical picture can occasionally appear in cases of hepatitis A, although only in one out of 10,000 cases. No effective therapy is available at this point that is directed against the virus itself. The present therapy is replacement of the liver by a transplant at the earliest possible moment.

Important note: Since the beginning of the 1980's a serum for the prevention of hepatitis B has been available. Many studies have proven its effectiveness. Those who are greatly at risk from hepatitis B are urgently advised these days to let themselves be inoculated.

No serum exists for hepatitis A, but in the short term, an injection of immune globulins has proven effective as protection against hepatitis A infections. For travel in high risk regions, such as Asia, preventive treatment with immune globulin is therefore recommended.

▶ *Liver Cirrhosis*

Today, the most common cause of liver cirrhosis is alcohol abuse. Alcohol as a toxic substance can cause an inflammation of the liver much like after a virus infection. Since during continued alcohol abuse the alcohol maintains the inflammation, it leads to the development of chronic hepatitis, which after a number of years can turn into a liver cirrhosis (from the Greek *kirrhos:* yellow, and *osis:* condition). The interval in which cirrhosis develops can differ. As their liver has a lower tolerance to alcohol, women develop cirrhosis more quickly than men. In the end, however, the pace at which the disease develops depends on alcohol consumption.

LIVER ENZYMES AND LIVER CIRRHOSIS   There is no liver-specific blood test to detect cirrhosis. No matter how helpful the measuring of liver enzymes is in monitoring acute and chronic hepatitis, it is of little use in indicating cirrhosis of the liver.

The development towards cirrhosis is gradual and hardly noticeable. The first symptoms are usually a feeling of tiredness and lack of energy. The progressive failure of liver functions leads to symptoms that are caused by other organs whose performance is being affected by the liver's diminishing ability to supply their needs.

Disruptions in hormonal balance occur: women stop menstruating, men develop a female breast shape, and the typically male distribution of body hair disappears. Increased tendencies toward hemorrhaging, fat metabolism disorders, and glucose metabolism disorders appear. Water is found in the abdominal cavity (ascites). A secondary circulation of blood drainage from the intestine via the esophagus forms (esophageal varices), and disruptions of the protein metabolism lead to ammonia poisoning of the brain. At this stage the damage to the liver is irreversible.

TUMOR MARKER ALPHA-FETOPROTEIN (AFP)   If a cirrhosis is present in conjunction with an infection with hepatitis B, and if the hepatitis serology (the lab tests for antigens and antibodies typical for hepatitis B) also detects the presence of HBSAG (hepatitis-B-surface-antigen), there is a significantly increased risk of developing liver cell carcinoma. In order to detect liver cell carcinoma as early as possible, AFP blood levels should be regularly monitored. In patients suffering from cirrhosis, the AFP level may already be increased slightly without signifying the presence of a liver cell carcinoma, so that progress monitoring, including annual tests of AFP levels is urgently advised for these high-risk patients.

If there is a significant increase in AFP levels, usually over 400 units per liter, further diagnostic methods, like computer tomography and/or ultrasound examinations of the liver have to be used to search very thoroughly for a liver cell carcinoma. Since liver cell carcinoma can occasionally be treated in its early stages by surgical procedures, early detection by monitoring of AFP levels is most important.

SUMMARY

Determining levels of the liver enzymes GOT and GPT is always of great importance when there is a suspicion of hepatitis. Transaminase levels that are elevated to several hundred units in conjunction with the clinical picture confirm a suspicion of hepatitis. A complete hepatitis lab test, including measuring levels of antibodies and antigens typical for the virus, helps to determine the cause and to classify the disease.

Liver enzymes can indicate a chronic hepatitis. If enzyme counts continue to be elevated six months after an acute hepatitis, a chronic hepatitis can be inferred. The transition from chronic hepatitis to a cirrhosis cannot be detected by determining transaminase levels. An AFP lab test can help to detect liver cell carcinoma in high-risk patients in time for therapeutic measures.

►► *The Gall Bladder—An Organ Rich in Stones*

Bile flows from our liver through the bile ducts into the duodenum. As a reservoir, our gall bladder is connected in parallel to the main bile ducts. It stores bile and concentrates it during fasting times. Hormones relate the message that food is being consumed, triggering contractions that cause the gall bladder to empty itself. Since our gall bladder is only a reserve storage organ we can actually live without it. If the gall bladder is removed our liver is able to adapt bile production to satisfy all our digestive requirements.

► *Diseases of the Gall Bladder*

Inflammations and stones can turn our gall bladder into a sick organ. Gallstones have become easier to detect since ultrasound examinations were introduced. They have enabled physicians to determine that the number of gallstone carriers who do not suffer complaints is much larger than had been thought. Especially those women who have had several pregnancies and who are overweight tend to be affected. This group contains up to 35 percent gallstone carriers, yet only 20 percent of them suffer any complaints.

FORMATION OF STONES The formation of gallstones depends on the composition of the bile. In industrialized countries, the stones most commonly encountered are cholesterol stones, whose formation depends on the cholesterol levels and bile acids in the bile. Normally both substances are in equilibrium, so that stone formation cannot be triggered. If cholesterol levels increase, or if bile acid concentration decreases, small bile crystals form, and over the course of months and years grow to become gallstones.

Gallstones can also develop due to increased destruction of red blood cells (hemolysis).

► *Blood Lab Tests Do Not Reveal Gallstones*

Among the routine lab test methods, none as yet can determine the presence of gallstones. Apart from general clinical factors, such as female gender, obesity, oral contraceptives, and predisposition due to family history, there is only the cholesterol level in the blood that can be used as a risk indicator for the formation of gallstones.

Similarly, an inflammation of the gall bladder (cholecystitis), which in most cases includes the presence of stones, cannot be confirmed by determining liver enzyme levels, even though there may be an increase in liver enzyme levels over the course of cholecystitis. This is, however, considered a sign of the liver's involvement in the inflammatory process.

SUMMARY

Elderly and overweight women have a high risk of developing gallstones. But by way of consolation, it seems that only 20 percent are likely to develop any painful complaints. It is not a problem to live without a gall bladder. Its diseases—gallstones and the inflammations that are frequently connected with them—cannot be detected by using blood tests. Our cholesterol level can be used as an indicator of the risk that gallstones may develop. The most useful test to detect the presence of gallstones is an examination using ultrasound.

►► *The Liver's Blood Clotting Agents*

To keep our blood flowing, on the one hand, and to enable it to close injured blood vessels, on the other hand, are the two tasks of the co-agulation equilibrium (hemostasis) in the blood. This equilibrium is maintained by balancing agents that aid clotting and those that prevent it.

A number of these clotting agents are produced in the liver. If the liver largely stops functioning, the concentration of necessary clotting agents in the blood will diminish. The resulting imbalance leads to coagulatory disorders. These become apparent through increased and prolonged menstrual bleeding, through extensive bleeding following minor injuries, through increased appearance of bruises, nosebleeds, and small, purplish, hemorrhagic spots on the skin which resemble fleabites (petechiae).

► *Thrombosis and Thrombolysis*

Currently there are 24 factors which, apart from platelets and calcium, are known to take part in this process (see clotting agents, above). Activating and inhibiting factors interlock in a cascading process in order to either form a sealing blood clot (thrombus), or to dissolve such a clot. The formation of a thrombus leads to thrombosis, its dissolving leads to thrombolysis. These two processes are constantly taking place in the body while an equilibrium is maintained between them. If thrombosis predominates it leads to arterial blockages, if thrombolysis dominates, bleeding occurs.

▶ *Blood Lab Tests for Liver Diseases*

Laboratory tests can detect many different clotting factors. For routine use, however, only a few such tests have proven useful on account of their ease of use and diagnostic capability. They record the clotting ability of the blood globally.

The test most commonly used to gain a quick overview is the determination of prothrombin time. It is used to record the most important clotting agents that are synthesized in the liver with the help of Vitamin K. A pathologically prolonged prothrombin time may be due to a deficiency in vitamin K levels, or to an insufficient ability of the liver to synthesize clotting agents.

The prothrombin time can therefore be used to show how far the liver's functioning is reduced. Abnormally prolonged prothrombin times are often found in connection with advanced liver cirrhosis, or in severe cases of hepatitis A as a sign of liver failure.

HEMOPHILIA A AND B   Hemophilia A and B are gender-dependent, congenital diseases of the blood coagulation apparatus. Since the disease is inherited by a defect in the female (x) chromosome, of which males have only one, men are more likely to develop hemophilia. The cause of the disease is a lack in blood clotting agents VIII (hemophilia A) or IX (hemophilia B). Depending on the levels of factors VIII or IX in the blood, a distinction is made between mild, intermediate, and severe forms of hemophilia. The lack of factors VIII (antihemophilic globulin) or IX (plasma thromboplastin cofactor) leads to an increase in the partial thromboplastin time (PTT). Less than one percent of factor VIII or IX in the blood, in conjunction with a family history of hemophilia, strongly suggests the presence of the disease.

VITAMIN K AND THE PROTHROMBIN TIME   Vitamins are considered "co-factors" for our body. The liver needs vitamin K in order to synthesize the factors known as the vitamin K-dependent factors, II (prothrombin), VII (proconvertin-Stuart), IX (plasma thromboplastin cofactor) and X (Stuart factor). Vitamin K is a fat soluble vitamin which the body cannot produce by itself, and which needs to be part of our diet. All fat soluble substances in our food can only be absorbed from the intestines into the blood with the help of bile.

If the flow of bile into the intestine stops, vitamin K can no longer be absorbed, and the liver can no longer produce the vitamin K-dependent factors. This is why a blocked bile passage or too little bile production in the liver leads to prolonged prothrombin time measurements.

COUMADIN® (WARFARIN) AND PROTHROMBIN TIME In the presence of medication that counteracts the effects of Vitamin K, prothrombin times increase. The length of the prothrombin time is used to fine-tune medication doses. Vitamin K antagonists (like Coumadin® are medications used as blood thinners in order to reduce the danger of thrombosis associated with certain diseases. Prothrombin times in patients being treated with this medication are often monitored in order to ensure that excessively large and excessively small doses are being avoided.

SUMMARY

In order to maintain hemostasis—the balance between thrombosis and thrombolysis in our blood—clotting agents are necessary. Important clotting agents are synthesized in our livers. A global lab test method for determining the functioning of hemostasis (clotting agent equilibrium) is the prothrombin time test. Since this test measures the agents that are produced primarily in the liver, it is also a good indicator of our liver's synthesizing performance. For patients being treated with Coumadin® the test is also used to monitor therapeutic success.

▶▶ Jaundice—The Disease That Turns You Yellow

Usually other people are the first to notice if someone is developing jaundice. First the whites of the eyes turn yellow, then the skin does, too. The stool changes color and the urine turns an ale-like brown. These symptoms indicate a case of jaundice (icterus).

Our liver produces bile whose yellow color is mainly due to the substance bilirubin. Bilirubin appears in our blood mainly when red blood corpuscles (erythrocytes) disintegrate. It is bound to albumin as a non-water-soluble substance, and in this way is transported through the bloodstream. As long as it has not yet been bound to certain transport substances (glucoronoids) in the liver cells it is called unconjugated (indirect) bilirubin. Once it has been resorbed by the liver cells, bilirubin is bound to the glucoronoids and released into the bile as conjugated (direct) bilirubin. Lab tests can distinguish between conjugated and unconjugated bilirubin.

▶ *Neonatal Jaundice*

A newborn's liver is not yet able to process bilirubin from the blood in sufficient amounts. After birth an increased disintegration of red blood corpuscles takes place, and there is an increased presence of hemoglobin (red blood pigment) which leads to an increase in indirect (non-bound) bilirubin in the newborn's blood. If the proportion of neonatal hemoglobin is particularly high, and if, therefore, a lot of bilirubin is present after birth, neonatal jaundice develops.

This can have toxic effects on the child's brain and lead to kernicterus. This is treated with ultraviolet radiation, and, in severe cases, by a blood exchange transfusion. The crucial factor in deciding which of these measures should be taken is the amount of bilirubin in the newborn's blood.

▶ *Jaundice Without Liver Disease*

Adults can also experience an increased disintegration of red blood corpuscles (erythrocytes). This process is called hemolysis. If hemolysis is very severe and affects more than a third of the blood's erythrocyte content, our liver cannot process the resulting inflow of bilirubin. Despite full resorption capability of the liver, the bilirubin level in the blood rises, resulting in a yellow coloring of the skin (icterus). In this case, however, the stool will not change color, since bile is still being excreted into the intestine.

These processes are usually triggered by transfusions of an incompatible blood type, by acute hemolysis, or by medication. In the presence of a certain congential enzyme deficiency (glucose-6-phosphate-dehydrogenase-deficiency), the risk of triggering hemolysis by certain medications is especially great. Hereditary causes of hemolysis include the large group of disorders referred to as hemoglobinopathies (abnormal hemoglobin disease). Amongst these is sickle cell disease, a single substitution in the gene controlling beta-globin synthesis. This causes cells to hemolyse, as well as to form rigid red blood cells which clog small blood vessels, leading to painful crises and organ disfunction.

▶ *Blood Lab Test for Hemolysis*

This form of icterus without liver disease is known as prehepatic icterus. The lab test shows a moderate increase in total bilirubin of up to 5 to 6 mg/dl, and a distinct increase in unconjugated bilirubin. In connection with an enzyme, lactatehydrogenase (LDH), and the bilirubin transport substance haptoglobin, lab testing can be used to detect prehepatic icterus.

LABORATORY TEST FOR HEMOLYSIS

Bilirubin (total)
Bilirubin (indirect)
Lactate dehydrogenase (LDH)
Haptoglobin

▶ *Jaundice (Icterus) and Liver Disease*

In connection with an inflammation of the liver (hepatitis), jaundice (icterus) can also develop. Due to an inflammatory reaction to either a virus infection or to the effects of alcohol, liver cells are compromised in their ability to conjugate and transport bilirubin, and bilirubin becomes congested in the liver cells. Another portion of the bilirubin cannot reach the gall capillaries by the usual path since the transportation mechanism of the liver cells is disrupted.

The result is a mixed increase of both conjugated and unconjugated bilirubin. The total bilirubin count in the blood can reach up to 30 mg/dl. Once the inflammatory reaction decreases, the icterus subsides after a few days' delay when compared to transaminase. At the same time, bilirubin drops to normal values.

Besides bilirubin, alkaline phosphatase (AP), and, if measured, gamma-glutamyl-transferase (GGT) values are also raised.

▶ *Blood Lab Test for Cholestasis*

AP and GGT (where applicable) are enzymes considered to be indicators of disruptions in bile production. During liver diseases such as hepatitis, but also during such chronic diseases as cirrhosis, blood levels of these enzymes are moderately elevated. Measurements increase until they reach up to 400 units, and then stabilize. These enzymes originate in the tissue that lines our bile ducts. They indicate that an inflammation is also affecting bile production in the liver. If over the course of a hepatitis signs of cholestasis increase, the hepatitis is called cholestatic hepatitis. This form appears especially in connection with the use of steroids or hormonal contraceptives.

Since disruptions in bile production are generally known as cholestasis these enzymes are our cholestasis indicators.

LAB TEST FOR CHOLESTASIS

Alkaline phosphatase (AP)
Gamma-glutamyl-transferase (GGT, gamma-GGT)
Bilirubin

Important note on medications and cholestasis markers: Cholestatic forms of liver disease often appear as side-effects of medications. As our detoxification organ, the liver is often affected by medication, and becomes involved in how they work on the body. Any form of liver damage—from an isolated inflammation to specific disruptions of bilirubuin-conjunction, to disruptions of transport mechanisms— can be caused by medication.

During treatment with hormones, anabolic steroids, psychoactive medication, pain killers, or barbiturates, it is important to repeatedly monitor the liver enzymes SGPT, SGOT, AP, and, where applicable, GGT, in order to detect side-effects in the liver as early as possible. Usually changes in blood values and liver function disappear once the medication is discontinued. In extreme cases, however, the use of such painkillers as Tylenol, or antibiotics like Tetracycline can lead to extremely severe disruptions of liver function. In order to monitor these therapies, especially if they continue over an extended period of time, it is urgently advisable to determine liver enzyme levels regularly. Ultrasound examinations are used to complement the lab monitoring.

ALCOHOL ABUSE AND GGT Gamma-glutamyl-transferase can be helpful in recognizing liver damage at an early stage caused by alcohol. If during testing an isolated increase in GGT is found without corresponding increases in AP and bilirubin, and if other causes have been excluded with certainty, a GGT value of 50 to 100 units in serum can point to alcohol abuse that has caused early stages of liver damage.

Usually there is a diagnosis of fatty liver, which can be confirmed by ultrasound or a liver tissue sample. After several weeks of abstinence from alcohol, both the increased GGT value and the fatty deposits in the liver may recede.

▶ *Jaundice (Icterus)—When the Bile Stops Flowing*

Bile drains from our liver in the bile ducts. The main stream of bile flows through a left and right bile duct from the liver, combining to form the main bile duct. If this passage is blocked the flow of bile stops completely. Bile no longer reaches the intestine, causing the stool to lose its normal tint and become clay-colored. The congestion of bile also increases the bilirubin level in the blood. If the blockage has been complete and has lasted long, values can reach up to 50 mg/dl. This is accompanied by a tormenting itch that affects the entire skin.

Even before an increase in bilirubin becomes measurable in the blood, the other cholestasis markers AP and GGT increase. They can reach values of more than 1,000 units. Values in this range are typical for diseases of the bile ducts. Thus it is possible from these signs together with an ultrasound examination of the bile ducts to discover if an occlusion of the bile ducts has occurred.

BENIGN AND MALIGNANT OCCLUSIONS There are essentially two possibilities that can lead to an occlusion of bile ducts. If jaundice is accompanied by attacks of colic, the reason is most likely a gallstone that has travelled from the gall bladder into the main bile duct and has there caused a benign occlusion.

If, on the other hand, icterus develops slowly and unnoticeably, and without the typical gall bladder colic, a malignant growth is blocking the bile duct. If this occurs in parts of the bile ducts that are situated towards the liver, there is usually a malignant tumor of the bile duct itself. Since these tumors are usually inoperable by the time they make themselves felt by an icterus, there is no curative therapy. Tumors next to the bile ducts which stem from the upper portion of the pancreas tend to close off bile ducts by external pressure on the section that is situated near the intestine. In these cases, too, the tumor has usually progressed too far for any therapy with a hope of curing the disease.

Recent developments in endoscopic techniques for the stomach, the intestine, and the bile duct have made it possible to reduce suffering. It has been a great help to relieve the itching sensation associated with bile duct blockages. This also means that the cosmetically bothersome yellow skin color disappears, and patients can once more gain confidence in their social contacts.

SUMMARY

There are many causes leading to jaundice (icterus). The main symptoms are yellow coloring of the eyes (scleral icterus) and of the skin, as well as clay-colored stool, and a dark brown color of the urine. Lab test results show an increase in bilirubin levels, from a typical 6 mg/dl in a prehepatitic icterus, up to 30 mg/dl in icterus involving liver disease, and up to 50 mg/dl in icterus involving occlusion of the bile ducts. Along with bilirubin, the enzymes and cholestasis markers alkaline phosphatase (AP) and gamma-glutamyl-transferase (GGT), are also increased to levels which can be as high as 1,000 units where there is icterus due to a blockage. With further lab testing one can determine whether it is a case of hemolysis (prehepatitic icterus) or of hepatitis (intrahepatitic icterus). If GGT alone is increased this points to fatty deposits in the liver due to alcohol.

7

STOMACH, INTESTINES, AND PANCREAS

Our stomach and intestines break down food so that it can be absorbed by our organism into the bloodstream for further processing. In the stomach there is both a mechanical and a chemical reduction of the food. Our pancreas produces digestive juices that help transform the three basic components of our food, carbohydrates, proteins, and lipids into a form that our body can use.

►► How Our Stomach, Intestines, and Pancreas Work Together: The Digestive Process

Our diet is composed of many different combinations of the above three basic substances. Potatoes, for example, consist mainly of starch. Starch in turn is composed of many thousands of sugar molecules that are strung together as in a chain. Food is transported through the esophagus, the stomach, and the small intestine into the large intestine, and its remains are from there excreted as stool. The combined contents of our intestines are a food paste and the secretions of our gall bladder and pancreas. Thus, every day several quarts of liquid intestinal content are formed to be processed by the intestinal mucous membrane. The most important function of the small intestine's membrane is to absorb carbohydrates, proteins, lipids, electrolytes, and vitamins. The water content is mainly ab-

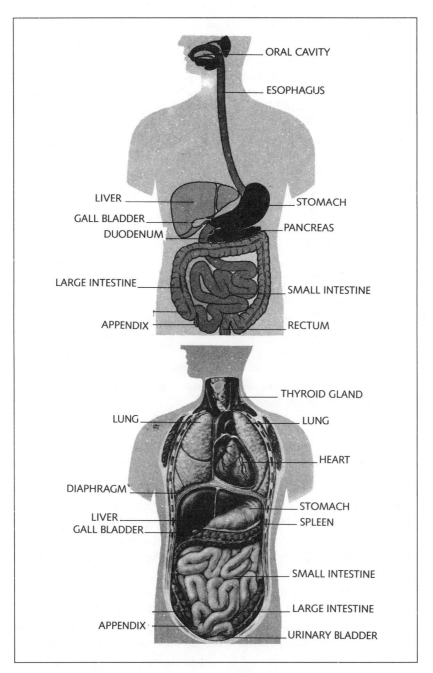

ORAL CAVITY

ESOPHAGUS

LIVER

GALL BLADDER

DUODENUM

STOMACH

PANCREAS

LARGE INTESTINE

SMALL INTESTINE

APPENDIX

RECTUM

THYROID GLAND

LUNG

LUNG

HEART

DIAPHRAGM

LIVER

GALL BLADDER

STOMACH

SPLEEN

SMALL INTESTINE

LARGE INTESTINE

APPENDIX

URINARY BLADDER

The digestive tract (above), and its position in the large body cavities (chest and abdominal cavity, below) sorbed in the large intestine. In this way on the several quarts in the small intestine are reduced to about 10 ounces (150 milliliters) that are excreted as stool every day. In order for the intestinal walls to be able to absorb carbohydrates, proteins, and fats, a food, like starch, has to be broken down in certain ways. This is the process we call digestion. If impaired digestion (malabsorption) occurs, our body can begin to suffer from various deficiencies. A main symptom of malabsorption is diarrhea, and it is due to an osmotic effect—the attraction to water of undigested sugary substances, such as milk sugar.

▶ Food Absorption

Disruptions of our stomach and intestines' absorption of the digested nutrients into the blood can be seen in the blood when a disruption (malabsorption) causes a deficiency in the levels of these substances. Lab tests can only roughly distinguish between functional disruptions in the large and the small intestines, since the large intestine has no significant capacity for absorbing nutrients. For example, the absorption of vitamin B12 occurs only in one narrowly defined section of the small intestine, the ileum.

Thus lab tests can be used to determine the extent, but not the causes, of absorption and digestive disorders. (Radiologic examinations and small bowel biopsies may be needed to define sites of malabsorption.)

▶ Digestive Juices from Our Stomach, Intestines, and Pancreas

In order to digest our food we require very large amounts (approximately 1½ gallons or 6 liters per day) of digestive juices (secretions). The main producers are our stomach, gall bladder, pancreas, and duodenum. While proteins are broken down in our stomach by acid as well as pepsin in addition to mechanical reduction, lipids and carbohydrates are broken down in the small intestine.

Our stomach acts like a cement mixer which moves the food paste in such a way that the solid food components are placed more in the center of the stomach, and the liquids are closer to the walls. In this way, liquid food components leave the stomach more quickly than solids, allowing more time for breaking down the latter.

► *Blood Lab Test for Poor Digestion*

If a digestive disorder has been present long enough, this leads to a lack in nutrients and to symptoms of deficiencies. Our blood transports all the nutrients that have been absorbed, and they can be detected by blood analysis. Where there is a deficiency, as, for example, in sugar, the result will be a low blood sugar level. For proteins and lipids the same holds true. Thus dysfunctions or diseases of the intestinal tract which cannot be detected by blood values typical for the intestine itself can be identified by a lack of nutrient substrates, such as lowered blood levels of sugar, protein, or lipids.

LAB TEST FOR DIGESTIVE DISORDERS

Albumin
Glucose
Calcium
Magnesium
Zinc
Folic acid
Vitamin B 12
Vitamin D
Cholesterol
Triglyceride

Important note: In searching for the causes of a digestive or resorption disorder it is best to use the methods of direct or indirect visual examination of the stomach and the intestinal tract. During these tests tissue samples can also be taken that are an important help in understanding what is causing the disease.

Indirect forms of examination with x-rays, especially of the stomach and intestines, are nowadays limited to the small intestine. Direct visual methods of examining (endoscopy) the stomach, the duodenum, and the large intestine have replaced x-ray examinations in these areas. Lab tests can only provide indications of abnormal processes in the search for the causes of digestive disorders.

SUMMARY

Our stomach, and small and large intestines are our digestive organs. There are functional differences between the digestion and absorption of nutrients into the blood. We differentiate between disorders of poor digestion and malabsorption. While our small intestine absorbs basic nutrients, electrolytes, and vitamins into the blood, our large intestine absorbs mainly water. The effects can be seen in the laboratory measurements. Information about the causes of intestinal disorders is gathered mainly by endoscopic and other imaging methods.

▸▸ *The Pancreas—The Largest Gland in Our Body*

Lipids, starch, and protein are digested and absorbed mainly in the upper region of the small intestine. The necessary digestive secretions are produced by our pancreas. With a daily production of more than three quarts it is the gland with the highest secretion output. Its structure is like that of the parotid gland in our lower jaw. Like the pancreas it secretes a digestive liquid 90 percent of which consists of an enzyme that can break down starch (amylase).

Our pancreas is functionally divided into two parts: a digestive part (exocrine pancreas) that produces digestive juices, and a hormonal part (endocrine pancreas, see *Diabetes,* p. 149) that controls our sugar metabolism.

▸ *Exocrine Pancreas*

Our exocrine pancreas forms a glandular secretion in the smallest gland particles (acini) that consists of enzymes to break down fat, protein, and starch. The most important enzymes are lipase, trypsin and amylase. The secretion flows by through drainage ducts into the duodenum. In order to create an optimal environment for the enzymes' activity our pancreas also secretes bicarbonate (alkaline solution). It helps to neutralize the acidic gastric juice that enters the duodenum, and to protect the duodenum's mucous membrane.

Lipase is able to break down fats, while trypsin breaks down protein, and amylase breaks down starch. Since all of these substances also occur as components of our own body tissues, nature has found a way of protecting our organism from destroying itself. The enzymes in question are produced in the gland as inactive preliminary substances, and are activated only once they have entered our intestines.

▶ *Diseases of the Pancreas*

Inflammations of the pancreas (pancreatitis) are always dangerous. There are two forms, acute and chronic pancreatitis. While the acute form is often responsible for a dramatic event in a person's life, the chronic form leads to long suffering, involving pain and weight loss.

ACUTE PANCREATITIS This usually appears as extreme pain that comes without warning after a good meal, waking the gourmet out of a deep sleep. Pancreatic pain—extreme pain in the middle of the abdomen below the sternum—is a characteristic sign. It can, however, be mistaken for an acute infarction of the heart's rear wall.

The cause for the inflammation is that digestive enzymes are secreted into the gland itself and into its surroundings. A variety of sensitive supply structures for our intestines, kidneys, spleen, and liver are situated near the pancreas. The fatty tissue which surrounds these neighboring organs is destroyed by lipase. Digestive substances similiar to those present in the normal digestive process are formed and can spread across the abdominal cavity and neighboring regions where they begin to digest our own body fat. The metabolic substances can trigger extreme reactions in other organs up to a state of circulatory shock.

Even today, the mortality rate for acute pancreatitis in its most severe form is 20 to 30 percent.

CHRONIC PANCREATITIS Lab tests for levels of pancreatic amylase or lipase cannot distinguish between acute and chronic inflammation of the pancreas. Only study of the clinical development can lead to a correct diagnosis.

During those stages of a chronic inflammation that are marked by attacks of pain, we often find elevated levels of pancreatic amylase and lipase, but in most cases these values are only a few hundred units, and therefore significantly lower than for an acute inflammation. However, if, apart from increasingly frequent pain episodes, there is a significant increase in lipase and amylase values, it is definitely necessary to initiate a further examination to reconfirm a diagnosis of chronic inflammation.

► *Blood Lab Test for Pancreatitis*

Laboratory tests are a valuable help in recognizing acute forms of pancreatitis. For chronic forms, on the other hand, tests are used only to detect the results of the chronic failure of pancreas function.

LAB TEST FOR PANCREATITIS

Lipase
Calcium
Amylase (p–Amylase)

LIPASE IN THE SERUM AS TRACING FACTOR When there are complaints of the type we have just described, a pathologically elevated lipase level in the blood permits a correct diagnosis. In cases of acute pancreatitis, lipase values can reach several thousand units. Where values exceed ten thousand units the prognosis is poor. An analysis of lipase levels can be the deciding factor in making the correct choice of diagnosis and therapy, particularly in distinguishing between pancreatitis and heart attacks. If both heart enzymes and lipase levels are measured, and if lipase levels are raised while heart enzyme levels are normal, the diagnosis of acute pancreatitis is certain.

SERUM CALCIUM—ITS SIGNIFICANCE FOR ACUTE PANCREATITIS In cases of acute pancreatitis a drop in serum calcium levels can often be detected. In severe cases serum calcium levels drop at regular intervals due to an inflow of blood-calcium into the inflamed tissue that surrounds the pancreas. As a result, calcifications occur which can later be seen in x-ray photographs as calcium shadows in the upper abdomen.

AMYLASE USED IN DIAGNOSTICS Up to a few years ago the most common method for diagnosing acute pancreatitis was to measure total amylase levels in the blood. There is, however, a special form of amylase—macroamylase—that can lead to elevated amylase levels even when pancreatitis is not the cause. Since the parotid gland can also secrete amylase, measuring amylase levels is not enough to determine with certainty if the pancreas is responsible for the pathological picture. Intestinal inflammations can also lead to raised amylase levels, because they increase the permeability of the intestinal wall and in this way mimic pancreatitc symptoms. In lab tests it has become a common practice to determine levels for pancreatic amylase, which is the variety of amylase that occurs only in the pancreas, since this allows for a greater degree of diagnostic precision, even when compared to lipase.

SUMMARY

Laboratory diagnostics are very helpful in cases of acute pancreatic inflammation. With certain levels of lipase and pancreatic amylase, certain typical complaints, pancreatitis can be diagnosed. It can be distinguished from acute cardiac infarct by, at the same time, measuring heart enzyme levels in the serum. Chronic forms of pancreatitis lead to a series of changes in lipase levels which can be judged confidently only where previous values are known.

►► *Tumors of the Pancreas, Stomach, and Intestines*

► *Pancreas Carcinoma—Often Detected too Late*

Only rarely is an attack of pancreatitis caused by a carcinoma of the pancreas—malignant tumor. The development of pancreatic carcinoma, a disease that tends to occur during the sixth decade of our lives, is usually painless during its early stages. When signs of the tumor appear, in the form of jaundice (icterus) or pain, it is usually too late for surgical therapy. The tumor has often grown to such a size that it cannot be removed entirely.

► *Tumors of the Stomach and of the Large Intestines*

Tumors of the stomach are appearing less frequently, but the same is not true for tumors of the intestines. The increase is due mainly to a larger number of colon carcinomas. There is also an increase in tumors of the large intestine in patients under forty. Laboratory diagnostics are not yet able to diagnose carcinomas of either the stomach or the intestine; both should be suspected when there is an iron deficiency anemia.

There are a number of tumor markers that can be measured in the laboratory, but none achieve diagnostic certainty. Certain symptoms, however, point toward a tumor in the stomach or in the intestines. Usually the development of both these forms of tumors is connected to a blood loss into the intestine. The number of red blood corpuscles and the hemoglobin content of the blood drop and anemia develops.

If the amount of blood lost in this way is less than 100 milliliters the color of the stool does not change. This invisible amount (also known as occult blood) can be detected by testing the stool. The test is conducted over the course of three days during which the patient must avoid eating raw meat and vitamin C supplements. Testing for occult stool blood is considered a screening test for cancer of the large intestine and is offered by many family doctors. If the results are positive even once, further tests must be conducted to determine the cause. In most cases the reason is not a carcinoma. Often, the cause is a peptic ulcer or intestinal polyp, although the latter can be a precursor to a tumor.

Important note: Endoscopy is the method of choice. Currently endoscopic methods of examining the stomach and large intestine are the safest ways to recognize tumors. Laboratory methods can be used to monitor the process of recovery, but endoscopy in conjunction with taking a tissue sample (biopsy) provides the confirmation for a suspected diagnosis.

Do not hesitate to ask your physician about endoscopic diagnosis of your stomach and intestines if the results of your physical examination or blood test (anemia) point toward a possible tumor.

▶ *Blood Lab Tests: Can Blood Tests Help Diagnose Cancerous Tumors?*

Only for certain types of cancer can indicators be found in the blood. These are known as tumor markers. For the most part they are complex proteins that are released from cancerous tissue into the bloodstream. A laboratory test can be used to detect elevated levels.

However, non-tumorous tissues can also produce these markers in increased amounts—for example, due to smoking or to inflammation. This means that tumor markers are not suitable for proving the existence of a tumor, even where high tumor marker levels lead to a suspicion of cancer. They are very useful, however for monitoring the progress of an existing tumor.

Pancreas carcinoma leads to an increase in CA 19–9.

Stomach and intestinal carcinomas, as well as breast cancer and lung carcinoma, lead to an increase in carcino-embryonic antigen (CEA).

MONITORING WITH THE HELP OF TUMOR MARKER CEA   Once a tumor has been diagnosed, carcino-embryonic antigen (CEA) is a valuable help in monitoring its development. In typical cases of intestinal carcinoma, before an operation, CEA levels in the blood are found to be elevated to a degree that reflects the tumor's extent. CEA is an expression of the embryonic dedifferentiation of tumor cells which are able to synthesize an increased amount of substances of the embryonic stage. This ability explains the term CEA.

TUMOR RECURRENCE IF CEA LEVELS RISE AGAIN   After an operation CEA levels drop to normal levels if the cancerous tissue has been removed entirely. As long as this normal level persists, recovery can be assumed. But if CEA levels rise above a certain limit, this usually indicates a recurrence of the tumor.

SUMMARY

Laboratory testing of the blood is not a suitable method for proving the presence of a tumor in the pancreas, stomach, or intestine. On the other hand, the effects of a tumor, such as anemia, can be easily recognized in the blood. However, even high levels of such tumor markers as CA 19–9 or CEA can only lead to the suspicion of a tumor. As with stool testing for occult blood, further diagnostic methods will be needed by your physician. Still, tumor markers are very useful in monitoring the development of known cancers.

Early diagnosis improves the chance for cure. If malignant tumors of either the stomach or the intestines are recognized early enough, chances of recovery are very good. This fact has caused some health insurance programs to offer coverage for preventive examinations of the large intestine.

8

THE KIDNEYS AND
URINARY BLADDER

Nature has provided us with two kidneys. Like a number of other functionally important organs, they are paired and placed symmetrically.

Both kidneys are well protected, toward the rear by the musculature of our back and by the bones of our spine, toward the front by our abdominal organs and muscles. The kidneys are situated in the retroperitoneal cavity. This is the anatomical area between the muscles of our back and the peritoneum, and bordering on the diaphragm where it extends towards the chest cavity. The tip of the left kidney is further protected by the left costal arch of our rib cage. This position explains why kidney diseases can lead to back pains that are often mistaken for complaints originating in the spinal column.

Our kidneys are the sole producers of urine. It is collected from many small channels in the pelvis of the kidney (renal pelvis) which radiates, glove-shaped, into the kidneys. From the renal pelvis our two ureters stretch over a distance of about eight inches (20 centimeters), until they reach the urinary bladder situated in the bony pelvis. In some people the length of the ureter is doubled.

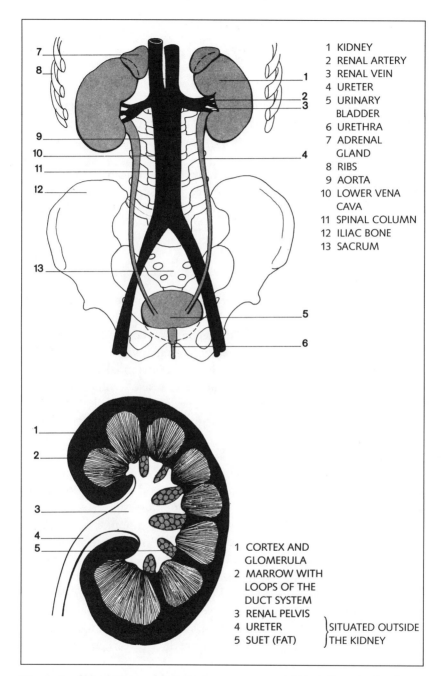

1 KIDNEY
2 RENAL ARTERY
3 RENAL VEIN
4 URETER
5 URINARY
   BLADDER
6 URETHRA
7 ADRENAL
   GLAND
8 RIBS
9 AORTA
10 LOWER VENA
   CAVA
11 SPINAL COLUMN
12 ILIAC BONE
13 SACRUM

1 CORTEX AND
   GLOMERULA
2 MARROW WITH
   LOOPS OF THE
   DUCT SYSTEM
3 RENAL PELVIS
4 URETER   } SITUATED OUTSIDE
5 SUET (FAT)   } THE KIDNEY

Diagram of the kidney and the urinary passages (above). Longitudinal section through kidney, kidney membrane, and renal pelvis (below).

▶▶ Bladder and Kidney Functions

▶ Our Bladder as the Control Organ for Urination

Our bladder is the basin which collects urine and controls its discharge. It can adapt to different amounts of urine of up to one quart (1 liter). However, excessive amounts of urine in the bladder cause severe pain, so that an overflowing urinary bladder is often associated with severe abdominal pain.

Urine is discharged from an opening at the bottom of the urinary bladder into the urethra. Using flexible endoscopic instruments we can visually examine (by cystoscopy) the urethra, urinary bladder, and the urinary ducts as far as the renal pelvis.

▶ Our Kidneys Regulate Their Own Blood Supply

Despite the fact that a single kidney weighs no more than 10 ounces (150 grams) its share of the blood supply at any time is about one quarter. By using a complicated mechanism controlled with hormones, our kidneys are able to regulate their own blood supply. In doing this they are not only the receptor of hormonal messages, but also the place where regulating hormones are synthesized. This double function allows them to independently control the rate of blood that flows through them (autoregulation of kidney blood supply).

The most important factor in kidney blood supply is blood pressure. In order to maintain blood pressure for their own supply, the kidneys take an active role in the body's blood pressure regulating system. They achieve this either by a hormonal system (renin-angiotensin system) or by directly controlling the amount of available blood. The renin-angiotensin system controls the blood pressure by affecting the resistance of the blood vessel walls. Thus, activating the system increases resistance while deactivating it decreases tension. Blood volume is controlled in the kidneys by an increase or decrease in urine production. These mechanisms enable our kidneys to maintain their most important function—blood filtration—independently of our other organ systems. The end product of this process is our urine.

URINE COMES FROM THE BLOOD   Blood filtration by the kidneys is like a chemical filter. Filtration takes place in the kidney corpuscles (glomeruli), where blood flows past a membrane that is permeable for certain substances. Two processes are at work in the glomerular filtrate. They are an active exchange of substances by pressure, and a passive exchange by osmotic diffusion. The permeability of the membrane is determined by its composition. The amount (volume) of glomerular filtrate depends mainly on blood pressure.

▶ Our Kidneys as Organs of Detoxification

The filtrate contains waste products from many different metabolic processes in our body. Thus, as well as our liver, our kidneys play a part in our body's metabolism. The kidneys also excrete toxic and foreign substances through the urine. Depending on the chemical composition of a substance like a medication drug, detoxification is carried out primarily by the kidneys or the liver. Substances composed of small molecules, and those known as heavy metals, like lead, are removed via the urine. If the amount of toxic substance exceeds the kidneys' capacity, the result can be kidney damage—analogous to liver damage—due to the accumulated deposits of the substance.

The total amount of filtrate produced daily is more than 40 gallons (170 liters). If this amount were actually secreted, it would quickly lead to a loss of so many important substances that we could only survive by being constantly connected to a pipeline supplying us with nutrients. But nature has seen to it that only one percent of the filtrate, about 1½ quarts (1½ liters) per day are actually secreted. The difference is reclaimed from the filtrate by our kidneys. This process, known as resorption, is possible because our kidneys contain a unique system of intertwining loops which are able to absorb water and substances that are dissolved in the filtrate back into the blood. By regulating such large amounts of liquid, our kidneys play a central role in our fluid equilibrium. They are in fact the central organ of our fluid equilibrium.

Since most of our body's electrolytes (sodium, potassium, calcium, and magnesium, as well as the hydrogen and bicarbonate that are important in our acid-alkaline balance) are dissolved in liquid, our kidneys also regulate our electrolyte equilibrium, and our acid-alkaline equilibrium.

▶▶ The Components of Urine

Nowadays most urine components can be analyzed in a laboratory. In the past, physicians based their observations about urine only on color, smell and—strange but true—taste. Today, a patient's urine analysis fills a large sheet of paper.

► *Sodium and Water*

By their volume, sodium and water are the two most important components of urine. The urine's volume and sodium content reflect the body's fluid equilibrium. If the concentration of sodium in the urine rises, and the amount of urine drops, the result is what we experience as thirst. Our kidneys reduce the amount of fluid secreted in order to conserve the body's water and a hormone (antidiuretic hormone) sends the corresponding signal to our kidneys.

Alcohol inhibits the function of this hormone—which explains why large amounts of alcohol in large amounts of liquid, as with beer, force us to urinate frequently.

► *Calcium*

One connection between our kidneys and the metabolism of our bones has been recognized only during the last twenty years. This is that the kidneys regulate our calcium balance both directly and indirectly. Bone consists mainly of calcium, which lends it hardness and strength. In cases of calcium deficiency the bone becomes brittle (osteoporosis). Our kidneys are involved in our bones' metabolism in two ways. They regulate the amount of calcium excreted into the urine; this can be easily confirmed by measuring the level of calcium in the urine. They also produce an important vitamin D hormone (1,25 vitamin D) which controls the formation of bone, and the absorption of calcium from food.

► *Protein*

The filtrate formed in the renal corpuscles (glomeruli) contains only small amounts of protein (up to 150 milligrams in 24 hours). The integrity of the glomeruli's membrane prevents larger amounts from passing through the barrier into the filtrate. But certain diseases change the membrane's permeability, and larger amounts of protein then appear in the urine. Simple urine test strip methods are useful for detecting concentrations of more than 500 milligrams. Thus, an increase in protein excretion is a sensitive measure for recognizing diseases of the kidneys and urinary ducts. Special analyzing methods can determine the protein's origin allowing us to locate the pathological process more precisely. It can also help determine if it is the kidneys or their secretion ducts that have been affected.

SUMMARY

Our kidneys and their secretion ducts form an integrated system for removing waste and toxic substances from the body. The kidneys are able to influence the equilibrium of our electrolyte, water, and acid-alkaline balance by means of various regulatory mechanisms. They also play an important part in regulating blood pressure and bone metabolism.

▶ *Blood Lab Tests: Is There Blood in the Urine?*

Though urine is formed out of blood, blood has no place in urine. Normally our blood is strictly separated from urine in our kidneys, renal pelvis, ureter, urine bladder, and urethra.

Just a few drops of blood are enough to stain urine noticeably red. However, other substances, like certain medications, can also lead to a red urine. In any case, a visible red discoloring of the urine due to blood (macrohematuria) is easy to recognize, and usually brings a person quickly into the physician's office.

A few single blood corpuscles (microhematuria), on the other hand, are visible only under a microscope. However, test strips are available which can indicate even invisible amounts of red blood corpuscles.

If blood appears in the urine it means that the barrier between the two substances has been breached somewhere in our body. This can happen in a number of places, and can occur anywhere along the urinary tract, wherever urine flows. Thus, damage in any location, from the kidney corpuscles (glomeruli) to the urethra can contribute to blood in the urine.

The presence of blood in the urine does not give us any information about its origin, and does not always support a diagnosis of kidney disease. Instead, it means that the entire urinary tract must be examined. The most common cause of blood in the urine is an infection of the lower urinary tract. Usually this is an inflammation of the bladder or the urethra. Kidney stones in the ureter can also lead to microhematuria, as can cases of colic. Finally, both benign and malignant growths of the urinary bladder can contribute to the presence of blood in the urine.

KIDNEY INFLAMMATION CAUSING MEMBRANE DAMAGE   Inflammations are the most common reason for changes in the glomeruli's membrane. If an inflammation is localized in the glomeruli it is called glomerulonephritis, or nephritis. Many forms of glomerulonephritis are originally caused by another illness. The best example is the once widespread kidney inflammations following scarlet fever and tonsilitis, in which the inflammation was the result of a remote infection with streptococci. Glomerulonephritis was not caused directly by these germs and none were found in the kidneys, but it was the result of defensive substances that had been formed against the germs.

If, as the result of an inflammation, membrane permeability is altered, up to 20 milligrams of protein can be secreted into the urine every day. In order to determine the exact amount, a test of urine collected over a period of 24 hours has to be conducted. Membrane damage due to inflammation can also increase the permeability of blood cells. Thus, kidney infections can make themselves known not only by an increase in protein secretion into the urine, but also by an increased number of red blood corpuscles in the urine (macrohematuria or microhematuria, depending on the amount).

WHY WE DO NOT TEST FOR BLOOD IN THE URINE DURING MENSTRUATION   The proximity of the openings of the urethra and the vagina means that during menstruation samples cannot be used to detect the presence of blood in the urine, unless the sample is taken with a urethral catheter. During menstruation there is always some blood present in the urine without it indicating a disease of the urinary tract.

THE IMPORTANCE OF COMPREHENSIVE TESTING WHEN THERE IS BLOOD IN THE URINE.   If lab testing of the urine leads to the detection of blood, a complete examination of the kidneys and urinary tract, including the urinary bladder, will be necessary. The only exception is for a woman during her menstrual period. If a negative microbiological urine test shows that there is no bacterial infection of the urinary ducts, then a comprehensive physical examination, and a complete analysis of the urine, especially for the presence of proteins, has to be made of the entire system of kidneys and urinary tract. It often becomes necessary to perform a visual examination (cystoscopy) of urethra and urinary bladder. This examination is further supplemented by x-ray diagnostics of the kidneys and their connecting ducts (excretion urogram) as well as by ultrasound examination of the kidneys. In men, an additional examination of the prostate is also urgently advised.

SUMMARY

Macro- and microhematuria are serious indicators of a urinary bladder and kidney disease. Detection is simple with the help of a test strip. Kidney inflammations lead to changes of the kidney filtration system which becomes permeable for proteins, so that elevated levels of protein (especially albumin) can be detected in the urine (proteinuria). If there is no bacterial infection of bladder or kidneys, further examinations beside a complete urine analysis will be needed.

▸▸ *When Our Kidneys Fail*

▸ *Acute and Chronic Kidney Failure*

If both kidneys fail this is a severe disruption of our entire organism. Because they are present in duplicate and because their function is safeguarded very well, our kidneys can maintain their function even under difficult physical conditions. But if severe circulatory disruptions (shock), severe infections (sepsis), or severe toxic damage due to poison occur, urine production stops (anuria) and acute kidney failure follows. If this state continues over several hours or days, the collecting of metabolic waste products leads to urine poisoning (uremia).

Before the days of mechanical blood cleaning (hemodialysis), people who suffered from this sickness died within a few days. Since machines for hemodialysis have become available, it has become possible for kidney function to recover after several weeks, once the remaining body functions have stabilized. For some patients, however, the outcome will be lifelong dependency on a dialysis machine.

In most cases, kidney failure develops gradually, over the course of several years. Most often it is due to recurring infections of the urinary tract (pyelonephritis) which ascend the ureter and affect the kidneys. A chronic process of shrinkage leads to scarring of the kidneys. The number of renal corpuscles contained in the kidneys decreases until blood filtration and the accompanying process of detoxification slowly come to a halt. This process is known as chronic progressive kidney insufficiency. Patients with this disease are almost certain candidates for machine dialysis. Kidney transplants have come to be frequently seen as a desirable alternative to mechanical kidney replacement therapy.

▶ *Blood Lab Test: Blood Values and Kidney Failure*

If the kidney's function as a filter decreases, there will be a rise in the levels of those substances that would normally be secreted by the kidneys into the urine. With chronic kidney failure these values rise slowly, and with acute kidney failure they rise quickly. A loss of up to three quarters of the normally present 1.2 million renal corpuscles can be compensated for by the remaining kidneys' detoxification performance, so that blood values do not rise.

Urine excretion is already disrupted at this point, even though values are still at normal levels, since under normal conditions the remaining glomeruli can compensate for the loss of the destroyed renal corpuscles' function. However, the fact that the remaining glomeruli are performing at the limit of their ability means that they cannot respond to any further increases in demand.

An inability to limit urine production even during periods of fluid deficiency, means that people suffering from early stages of kidney insufficiency pass large amounts of urine, even during periods of thirst. This often becomes apparent in the urine's straw yellow color, and in an increase in nighttime urine production. An increase in volume also causes fluid to collect in other parts of the body (edema), such as in the face, or in the ankles.

THE RETENTION VALUES   If the kidney insufficiency continues to progress, changes in blood values soon become apparent in lab testing. As important waste products are retained in the blood instead of being secreted into the urine, they are referred to as retention values. Blood urea nitrogen (BUN) can no longer be eliminated from the protein metabolism, creatinine cannot be eliminated from the creatinine metabolism (metabolism of the muscles), and both blood values increase, by about the same amount.

Since the creatinine value is dependent on muscle mass which varies from person to person, blood urea nitrogen values are used as a marker for the disruption of kidney functions. As a rule, blood urea nitrogen levels of more than 200 mg/dl indicate an acute case of insufficient urine production, and the necessity of using a machine for blood filtration. In cases of chronic kidney failure, the retention values in conjunction with clinical signs, such as the patient's general state of health and disruptions in other organ functions determine if mechanical therapy should be used.

RETENTION VALUES

Blood urea nitrogen (BUN)
Creatinine

ELECTROLYTE METABOLISM AND ACID-ALKALINE EQUILIBRIUM
The electrolytes sodium and potassium are important measuring parameters for judging the extent of kidney failure. While our organism is able to maintain sodium secretion at tolerable levels for some time, disruptions in blood potassium levels become noticeable much more quickly. If potassium levels are too high, our organism quickly reaches the limits of its tolerance and disruptions in the heart rhythm result. Once blood potassium levels rise above 6 mmol/l, the risk of a deadly disruption steadily increases. Values of more than 6.5 mmol/l in patients with kidney failure mean that mechanical dialysis must be used, as well as other means to reduce serum potassium.

The accumulation of positively charged hydrogen ions causes an increase in the blood's acidity. Apart from our kidneys, our lungs are the only organ able to influence the acid-alkaline equilibrium. An increasing imbalance towards acidity in the blood leads to a disruption of muscle function (muscle cramps). In the end, enzymes that are necessary for all vital functions can no longer perform their task. The unit of measurement for the acid-alkaline equilibrium is the pH-value. It is measured on a scale ranging from 0 to 14, with 7 being the central value at which acids (0–7) and alkalis (7–14) neutralize one another. The lower the pH value, the more acidic a substance is, the higher the pH value, the more alkaline (or basic) it is.

In our blood, a normal or neutral value is 7.4. If it drops below 7.2 this means severe overacidification (acidosis). This disruption can be corrected effectively by mechanical dialysis.

ERYTHROPOETIN When patients suffer from chronic kidney failure their appearance usually provides the first clue to the disease. Kidney patients often have a pale-yellow skin tint. One reason for this is anemia. After a prolonged kidney insufficiency, blood hemoglobin values drop to as low as 5 mg/dl. This anemia is not the result of blood loss but of a shortage in blood production.

Our kidneys produce the hormone erythropoetin, which is important in blood formation. Chronic kidney insufficiency leads to a shortage of this hormone, causing anemia. Blood formation comes to a halt while erythrocytes continue to be broken down at the normal rate or even at an accelerated rate. The result is a gradual decline in blood hemoglobin. Today, the synthetic production of erythropoetin makes it possible to treat anemias due to kidney insufficiency.

OTHER BLOOD MEASUREMENTS Apart from these disruptions in blood composition which, in cases of chronic kidney failure, often require constant monitoring, there are also other changes in the blood. Usually calcium metabolism is affected and the blood's calcium level drops while the phosphate content rises. The hormonal balance shifts, involving an increase in the parathyroid hormone (parathormone) and a decrease of vitamin D. The blood's insulin content rises as well as the hormone, gastrin, that increases the production of stomach acid. Thus kidney insufficiency leads to a large number of changes in the blood values.

LAB MEASUREMENTS FOR MONITORING OF CHRONIC KIDNEY FAILURE

Blood urea nitrogen (BUN)
Creatinine
Sodium
Potassium
Calcium
Phosphate
Blood picture

Important note: Since a number of medications are eliminated from our body by the kidneys, it is important to know if kidney insufficiency is present. If medication is taken in inappropriate amounts during kidney insufficiency, it may accumulate to dangerous levels. Side effects also appear more frequently if an excessively high amount of these substances remains in the blood. Blood measurements have been developed for particularly dangerous forms of medication. The limited therapeutic range of these medications, for example digitalis, means that their intake by patients with kidney insufficiency must be monitored with extreme care.

SUMMARY

Acute and chronic kidney failure means a loss of the kidneys' function of secretion. Reduction in urine volume leads to an accumulation of metabolic waste products in the body, which can culminate in urine poisoning. As kidney function is reduced, the retention values of blood urea nitrogen and creatinine rise proportionately. Relative values in electrolyte balance and in the acid-alkaline equilibrium also change. The results are increased levels of potassium, lowered calcium values (hypocalcemia), and anemia. In addition to clinical examination, the patient must be monitored by means of laboratory tests.

9

OUR ENDOCRINE SYSTEM

Without our system of hormone glands, our ordered vital body processes would be impossible. Our entire system is organized according to the principle of hormonal control of biological processes. The task of our hormone glands is to produce and secrete whatever hormones they each specialize in. They form a unique system of communication within our organism. This is why hormones are also referred to as messenger substances.

One visible sign of how pervasive our network of hormonal control is, can be seen in the placement of the hormone glands, which are distributed throughout our entire body. We can find hormone-producing glands in our brain, in our neck, in the abdomen, in our retroperitoneum, and in the genitals. Many organs, in addition to their primary function, also play a role in our inner secretion system. The heart, for example, produces a hormone (the natriuretic factor) that increases kidney function—while our kidneys secrete a hormone (erythropoetin) that stimulates red blood cell formation.

►► How Hormone Glands Work

Our entire system of hormone glands is also known as the inner secretion system (endocrine secretion). Thus, tissues that are capable of producing hormones secrete these into the blood circulation, in con-

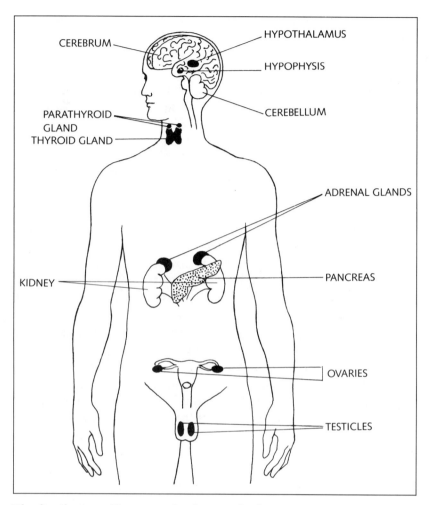

CEREBRUM

HYPOTHALAMUS

HYPOPHYSIS

CEREBELLUM

PARATHYROID GLAND

THYROID GLAND

ADRENAL GLANDS

KIDNEY

PANCREAS

OVARIES

TESTICLES

The distribution of hormone glands in our body

trast to the exocrine secretion performed by the sweat glands, or the pancreas, which secrete their substances either to the outside or into body cavities. Hormones reach their target location mainly by being transported in the blood. However we now know that nerve tracts and the fluid between cells (interstitial fluid) are also used to exchange hormonal messages.

These discoveries regarding the connection between hormones and nerve tracts have led to the development of a new branch of medicine—neuroendocrinology. It deals with the mutual effects of nervous system and hormonal messages. One field of research that has been publicized even in the popular press is the study of endorphines which are intermediary substances that control certain brain functions.

The knowledge that hormones are being transported in our blood has stimulated laboratory medicine to research this area. Consequently the research into the endocrine system has concentrated on detecting hormones in the blood by means of laboratory chemical and radioisotope methods.

▶ *How Hormone Secretion is Controlled*

Determining the concentration of individual hormones is essential for diagnosing disruptions of the inner secretion. These measurements can be accurately interpreted only with an understanding of how our hormones are controlled and how they function. We understand the regulatory mechanisms and routinely measure those hormones that are well-known. They work on the principle of negative feedback, where a feedback cycle regulates the secretion of the hormone based on its concentration in the blood or interstitium.

One example of this is the thyroid hormone. It is produced in the thyroid gland and is secreted into the bloodstream from there. If there is a pathological increase in the thyroid hormone's blood level, this triggers a reduced production of another hormone (TSH) whose role it is to stimulate thyroid production. This continues until thyroid hormone levels have returned to normal.

In order for such negative feedback loop mechanisms to function, superior coordination centers are necessary. Thus, our hormonal system is divided into a hierarchy of "superior" and "inferior" hormone glands. The relationships by which they affect one another are referred to as axes. Important hormonal axes in our body are the hypothalamus–hypophysis–thyroid axis, and the hypothalamus–hypophysis–adrenal cortex axis. In both of these, control signals are sent from the brain (hypothalamus) via the hypophysis to the hormone glands in the neck (thyroid), or to the adrenal cortex.

▶ *How Hormones Function*

Hormones are messenger substances. They create action from a distance. The hormonal glands from which they stem are not involved in their effects; instead their effect is provided by their target organs or tissues. Among the cells of the target organ there is a system of effectors. Since a single hormone can have different effects in different cell systems, nature has devised a sophisticated system of receptors. Receptors act like locks which need the right key (hormone) in order to open the door. By the specific nature and shape of the receptors on its different tissues, each organ receives the specific message that triggers the hormone's effect. Thus, insulin acts on our muscle tissue by triggering the resorption of glucose as a carrier of energy, while the very same hormone acts on liver cells by effecting the synthesis of glucogen (starch) for energy storage.

▶▶ *Diabetes—A Disease You May Not Know You Have*

Diabetes mellitus is a disease in which the connection between a hormone deficiency and its effects has been known for almost a hundred years. This connection is a typical sign of an endocrine disruption.

It is estimated that more than one percent of the populations of Western countries are suffering from diabetes melitus. More precise figures are unavailable, since a large portion of the population does not know that they are suffering from the disease. Moreover, it has only been a few years since the World Health Organization (WHO) has defined a set of criteria by which the disease can be assessed. The discovery of patients who do not know that they have diabetes is the main challenge of laboratory tests. Mass examinations to detect sugar in the urine have already shown that this method can be used to find those who have not yet developed any complaints.

▶ *How Does Diabetes Mellitus Develop?*

The cause of diabetes mellitus is a hormone disruption. Its effect is a disruption of the body's entire metabolism.

The most important hormone for our glucose metabolism is insulin, which is produced in the pancreas' beta-cells. These are also known, after their discoverer, as Langerhans cells. They are located mainly in the pancreas' tail section. Insulin-producing cells, and the alpha-cells which produce glucagon (another hormone which takes part in the sugar metabolism), are referred to as the endocrine pancreas, in contrast to the exocrine pancreas. If the beta-cells can no longer produce sufficient amounts of insulin, or if the effect of insulin on organs such as our musculature and liver is reduced, diabetes mellitus develops.

TWO FORMS OF DIABETES MELLITUS In the development of diabetes mellitus, there are two types: type I, insulin-dependent diabetes, and type II, insulin-independent diabetes. In young people insulin-dependent diabetes, which according to our current understanding constitutes an immunological disease, is more common. Insulin-independent diabetes, which occurs more often and usually in adults, is linked to a genetic predisposition. The first type means that insulin must be supplied to the body, while the second type is treated initially with medication, as well as with dietary measures.

▶ *Blood Lab Test for Diabetes Mellitus*

TESTING FOR SUGAR IN THE URINE Diabetes was already known to physicians in antiquity, who noted that the patient's urine tasted sweet. Today, the quick way of detecting sugar in the urine is the test strip method. An increase in sugar excretion can be recognized by the color change in a test strip. This method works well for testing large numbers of people, as well as for testing one's own urine at home. But since urine sugar levels vary, this method is not very exact. After a meal that is rich in carbohydrates, a healthy person's urine can also contain sugar.

BLOOD SUGAR MEASURING This is the more reliable method. If the blood glucose level after a twelve hour fast and on two consecutive days is higher than 140 mg/dl, a diabetes mellitus is present. It is usually the insulin-independent type. For further monitoring, regular glucose measuring is necessary. These controls also require that several blood value measurements are taken over the course of a day to draw up a daily blood sugar "profile." This profile shows whether the therapy (medication and/or diet) is successful in keeping blood sugar values in the normal range, and if it prevents blood sugar peaks throughout the day. It also provides information about the degree to which the metabolic disorder is under control.

Another lab measurement which is used to assess the metabolic situation is Hemoglobin A_{1C} (Hb A_{1C}) which is the proportion of a minor fast-moving hemoglobin in the blood. If this value is too high, it points towards a long-term disruption in the sugar metabolism. These long-lasting disruptions in sugar metabolism lead to the most serious consequences of diabetes, such as diseases of the retina, kidneys, and blood vessels.

THE GLUCOSE TOLERANCE TEST If individual blood sugar tests

have not led to a clear picture of the diabetic metabolism, one option is the glucose stress test. This is a test of the body's reserves in compensating for certain metabolic imbalances.

In the glucose tolerance test, the patient is given 5 ounces (75 grams) of glucose to drink. Blood samples are taken every thirty minutes for the first two hours after the sugar has been consumed, to determine blood sugar values. A healthy sugar metabolism is able to quickly break down this highly concentrated sugar solution by proportionately increasing insulin production. In a dysfunctional sugar metabolism, initial blood sugar levels will be higher than 200 mg/dl, and after two hours they will still remain between 140 mg/dl and 200 mg/dl. If all measurements, including the value after two hours, are higher than 200 mg/dl, this indicates diabetes mellitus.

METHODS FOR DETECTING DIABETES MELLITUS

Urine sugar (test strip method)
Blood sugar
Oral blood sugar tolerance test

▶ *Lab Methods for Controlling Diabetes Mellitus*

HYPOGLYCEMIA (LOW SUGAR) During insulin therapy for diabetes mellitus, hypoglycemia can occur. It is distinguished by hunger attacks, agitation, and disrupted consciousness. The suspected diagnosis should be immediately confirmed by a blood test. Blood sugar levels of less than 50 mg/dl strongly suggest a hypoglycemic state. The therapy consists of an immediate supply of glucose.

INSULIN PRODUCING TUMORS In a few rare cases, insulin producing tumors (insulinomas) are responsible for hypoglycemic states. Simultaneously measuring blood glucose and blood insulin levels may help to confirm this diagnosis, suspected because these tumors produce insulin independently of the body's glucose requirements. Normally, since our glucose requirements are reduced during fasting, blood insulin levels are also low. If a patient with an insulin-producing tumor is made to fast (fasting test), insulin levels will be normal, or even elevated, despite a fasting blood glucose level. This helps prove that increased insulin secretion is taking place, independent of blood glucose values. This fasting test must be conducted only on in-patients. Therapy for insulinoma consists of surgical removal of the tumor.

LABORATORY VALUES FOR MONITORING DIABETES MELLITUS

Blood sugar day profile

Hb A_{1C} (hemoglobin level)

SUMMARY

Diabetes mellitus is a metabolic disorder which manifests itself in raised blood glucose levels, and by an increased secretion of sugar into the urine. Its cause is either a lack of insulin or a decreased effect of insulin on the body's tissues. These disruptions are easy to measure with modern laboratory methods. If measuring blood glucose levels during fasting is not sufficient to confirm a diagnosis of diabetes mellitus, it is possible to conduct an oral glucose tolerance test. In order to monitor diabetes mellitus therapy, several blood glucose measurements are taken throughout the day (blood sugar daily profile), and Hb A_{1C} (hemoglobin) is measured.

▶▶ The Thyroid Gland and Hormones

Our thyroid is a small gland which is normally hidden beneath the larynx. It consists of a right and left lobe weighing less than an ounce (only a few grams) apiece. In some areas of the world, thyroid disease is the most common disruption of the endocrine system. This is because a lack of iodine leads to frequent incidences of goiter.

▶ Iodine as a Building Block of Thyroid Hormones

Iodine is needed for the production of thyroid hormones. Our thyroid is the only organ that can accumulate and store iodine. Thus, iodine concentrations in the thyroid tissue are forty times higher than those in the blood. Thyroid cells produce a protein (thyroglobulin) which is used as a transport and storage protein within the thyroid. The thyroid hormones T3 and T4 are also bound to it. If demand increases, a part of what was bound to the thyroglobulin is used as a reservoir and secreted into the bloodstream. The largest proportion is Tetraiodothyronine (T4), and it is transformed in the tissues of different organs. In the liver, for example, it becomes Triiodothyronine (T3). This is why it is usually necessary to replace only the T4 hormone during thyroid therapy which involves medication. The names of these hormones indicate the number of iodine atoms that are bound to every one of their molecules: three in one case, four in the other. In our blood, thyroid hormones are bound to a carrier substance, thyroxin-binding globulin (TBG). Lab tests can identify T3, T4, and TBG.

IODINE DEFICIENCY AND GOITER FORMATION   We normally require between 150 and 300 milligrams of iodine per day. Different geographical regions have different levels of naturally occurring iodine, and the closer to the ocean, the more iodine is present. This means that in some areas there is less iodine in normal foods than is needed to supply thyroid hormone production. To compensate for iodine deficiency, the thyroid gland increases its hormone production. An increase in production leads to an increase in mass, and this is the first stage in the formation of goiter. If a patient bends back the head and swallows at the same time, it usually becomes visible in the shape of a round bulge. If the iodine deficiency continues, the thyroid enlarges further, and parts of it are transformed into nodules. This stage is known as nodular goiter. During the first stage, a goiter can be reversed by increasing iodine supply. This is the reason why in some countries, as in the U.S.A. and Canada, iodine supplements are mandatory in table salts.

THE REGULATION OF THYROID HORMONE PRODUCTION   Goiter formation is directly connected to the regulatory mechanism of hormone production. The part of our brain known as the hypothalamus forms a hormone (TRH), which triggers the secretion of thyreotropin in the hypohysis (TSH), which in turn controls thyroid gland production and the thyroid gland's growth rate. TSH can be detected in the blood. If T3 and T4 increase TSH decreases, and the reverse.

▶ *Blood Lab Tests for Thyroid Function*

TSH AS A FUNDAMENTAL VALUE   To test the level of thyroid hormone production it is usually enough to determine TSH levels in the blood. This is done with a highly sensitive and precise TSH test (s—TSH). Under normal conditions the amount of TSH in the blood will reflect an excess or deficiency of thyroid hormone according to their relationship in a regulatory feedback loop. Hormone substitutes given orally can also be monitored by measuring TSH levels.

LABORATORY TESTING OF THYROID FUNCTION

Triiodothyronine (T3)
Tetraiodothyronine (T4)
s—TSH

EXCESSIVE AND REDUCED THYROID FUNCTION   A thyroid hyperfunction (hyperthyroidism) is present if more thyroid hormones circulate in the bloodstream than are necessary for the needs of our organism. Since only that part of the hormone which is not bound to the carrier protein TBG is important in its effect on our organs, a quantitative measurement of hyperthyroidism is made from free T4 (f—T4) hormone. The two measurements, TSH and f—T4, are useful in detecting nearly all disruption of the thyroid hormone metabolism.

SUMMARY

Goiter is a disease of the thyroid gland, and is a result of iodine deficiency. It appears more frequently in geographical regions with naturally low levels of iodine in food and water. The thyroid gland produces the hormones T4 and T3, but only T4 is secreted into the bloodstream. If blood levels for these hormones are elevated they can indicate thyroid hyperfunction. If they are depressed, they indicate thyroid hypofunction. A simple laboratory value to be used for both thyroid diagnostics and for monitoring thyroid therapy is the hypophysis hormone s—TSH.

►► *Adrenal Glands and Stress Hormones*

► *Adrenal Glands Are a Chemical Factory*

Humans have two small glands that are located near the upper poles of our kidneys, and are known as the adrenal glands. They weigh less than an ounce (only a few grams). The hormones they produce constitute a richly varied system of chemical substances. These hormones take part in many different processes throughout our body. The spectrum of their effects ranges from influencing inflammation reactions to affecting our sugar metabolism (glucocorticoids), from sexual development, blood pressure, heart rate, and fat metabolism (catecholamine), all the way to influencing our electrolyte balance (mineral corticoids).

Anatomically we distinguish between the adrenal cortex (outer rim) and the adrenal medulla (inmost portion or "marrow"). The adrenal medulla produces catecholamines, while the adrenal cortex synthesizes mineral- and gluco-corticoids.

THE REGULATION OF STRESS HORMONES   The adrenal medulla's activity is regulated via the nerve tract. There is a feedback mechanism for the activity of the adrenal cortex which we understand at least in principle. As in the thyroid gland, our brain, hypophysis, and adrenal cortex form a common regulatory mechanism. The brain's substances (the corticotropin-releasing hormone, CRF) increases the hypophysis' hormone corticotropin (ACTH), which, in turn, triggers the secretion of cortisol from the adrenal gland.

THE IMPORTANCE OF STRESS HORMONES   The catecholamines and corticoids are our stress hormones. They become significant when our organism is stressed. They are secreted in large amounts. They prepare our body for an increase in energy production and for a more efficient use of the available energy reserves. The secretion rhythm of cortisol was the first indicator of a daily biorhythm in our endocrine glands. Thus, the concentration of cortisol is highest at 4 a.m. and lowest at 2 p.m. Knowledge of their individual circadian rhythms is an important factor in judging hormone levels.

► *Blood Lab Test for Adrenal Gland Function*

The adrenal cortex produces a large variety of substances which are grouped into corticosteroids, mineral corticoids, and to a lesser extent, sex hormones. The main protagonists of these subgroups are, among the corticosteroids, cortisol, from the mineral corticoids, aldo-sterone, and among the sex hormones, testosterone and estrogen. (See *Our Sex Hormones,* below.) All of these substances can be detected in the blood with lab test methods. The regulating substances CRF and ACTH can also be detected in the laboratory. This means that, from the lab chemical point of view, we can record nearly all of the adrenal cortex's functions.

LABORATORY TEST OF ADRENAL GLAND FUNCTIONS

Fasting cortisol
Dexamethasone suppression test
Aldosterone

ADRENAL HYPO- AND HYPERFUNCTION   When excessive amounts of cortisol are produced they trigger an adrenal gland hyperfunction (the Cushing syndrome). This disruption can originate either in the hypophysis (increased ACTH production), or in the brain (increased CRF production). In both cases the adrenal glands increase in size, and detectable tumors develop. The typical daily rhythm of secretion is suspended. More and more waste products of the corticoid metabo-lism are found in the urine. The patient's appearance also changes with an increase in fat accumulation on the trunk. Due to the many effects of cortisol, diabetes mellitus, fat metabolic disorders, hyper-tension, and electrolyte balance disruptions develop.

With hypofunction cortisol production falls below a critical level. The result is a depressed cortisol blood level and a decrease in the amount of waste products secreted into the urine. If the disruption is due to a loss of the hormones CRF or ACTH, for example, due to inflam-mation of the brain or to a tumor, their blood levels will also be de-pressed. By measuring the levels of ACTH and CRF we can differentiate between central organic and glandular disruptions. This hypofunc-tion is known as Addison's disease.

If cortisol is lacking, stress reactions of the body can lead to a breakdown in energy supply balance. If this happens the organism is in mortal danger.

The most frequent cause for such conditions as Cushing syndrome is an overdose of corticoids as medication. Corticoids have greatly enriched the therapeutic spectrum of medicine, but large doses cause the same symptoms as a pathological disruption in adrenal cortex function.

SUMMARY

Adrenal cortex hormones and adrenal medullary hormones are also known as stress hormones. The adrenal cortex's hormones are mainly corticoids, especially cortisol. It also produces aldosterone, and to a lesser extent sex hormones. These hormones can be measured in the lab. This is how the two most important diseases, Cushing syndrome and Addison's disease, can be diagnosed via hormone analysis.

▸▸ *Our Sex Hormones*

Testosterone, estrogen, and progesterone are our sex hormones. They are a family, not only because of their common function, but also because of their common ancestry. The most important production takes place in the sex glands of the testicles and ovaries, respectively, and to a lesser extent the adrenal cortex. As their effects are easily visible they were the first hormones to be studied scientifically.

The most important functions of our sex hormones are the development of our secondary sex characteristics (pubic hair, and development of the female breast), and enabling sexual reproduction.

Every hormone production is regulated by a complicated feedback mechanism. Sex hormone production is also controlled, by our brain. The hypothalamus, in response to the amount of sex hormones in the blood, secretes a trigger hormone (luteotropin-hormone-releasing-hormone, LHRH) which affects the hypophysis. The secretion of LHRH is influenced by drugs, for example opium derivates, and by stress factors (via stress hormones). This explains why these influences can cause changes in our sexual behavior.

▸ *What Causes Our Development into Males and Females?*

The development of the fetus into a boy or girl occurs as early as the first weeks of gestation in the womb. Nature seems to have given priority to the development of female organisms, since an undisturbed process of development of sexual differentiation results in a female child. Only in the presence of sufficient amounts of inhibiting testosterone does the male type develop. The impulse for a sufficient amount of testosterone to be present at the critical moment is triggered by the male genetic constellation (XY chromosome). In the female genetic constellation (XX chromosome) this genetic information is suppressed. Gene-technological experiments on the chromosomes (XX and XY) of mice have shown that it is possible to control the sexual differentiation of their offspring.

Testosterone measurements in the mother as a means of determining whether a child will be male or female, however, is not useful. Hormone concentrations in the unborn are too low and cannot be detected in the mother's blood or urine. But it is now possible to identify the child's gender with ultrasound imaging at the end of the sexual differentiation period (twelfth week approximately).

▶ *Puberty—A Hormonal Event*

In terms of our hormone metabolism, our childhood prior to puberty is a kind of "sleep." Boys and girls have sex-specific hormones (testosterone in boys, estrogen in girls), but their levels are very low. As well the controlling hormones in the brain and hypophysis are not yet being secreted in the typical patterns.

The beginning of puberty is initiated by the appearance of the typical male and female biorhythms in the central hormone secretion. Hormone peaks of LHRH occur, and under their influence the hypophysis secretes larger amounts of luteotropic hormone (LH) and follicle stimulating hormone (FSH). These hormones cause maturation of the secondary sex characteristics, and hormone production in the sex-specific glands. In men these are the testicles, in women they are the ovaries.

▶ *Biorhythms and Menstruation in Women*

The production of sex hormones in our sex glands follows a day-and-night rhythm. The concentrations of testosterone and estrogen are highest in the morning and lowest during the late afternoon.

A typical example of a biorhythm is the periodic menstruation of women. Despite the fact that in individual women fluctuations of a few days are possible, the periodic appearance of menstrual bleeding is a firm biological rhythm that is typical for the female gender. The regular monthly bleeding is determined by the hormones estrogen and progesterone. A regular menstruation cycle is therefore also an important sign of regular hormone secretion, which takes place in the ovaries during regular menstruation.

▶ *Love and Pregnancy—Captivated by Hormones?*

Without the effects of our sex hormones there would probably be no such thing as love, and certainly no successful reproduction. In both men and women the ability respectively to procreate and to conceive depends on an intact system of sexual hormone production. The production of male sperm cells in the testicles is only possible under the influence of testosterone. The growth of the female egg for fertilization in the ovaries is possible only in the presence of a regular hormone cycle. Pregnancy and the gestation of a child is also only possible due to the protective functions of the hormones progesterone and estrogen.

▶ *Blood Lab Tests for Sex Gland Function*

MONITORING OF PREGNANCY BY ESTROGEN MEASUREMENTS The viability of a pregnancy can be monitored by measuring estrogen levels in the urine. If the values are too low for a particular pregnancy week, and if other factors indicate a danger to the child, a birth by cesarian section may have to be considered.

LABORATORY TESTS OF SEX HORMONES

Hypophysis hormone LH–FSH
Estrogen
Testosterone

HORMONE LABORATORIES AS FERTILITY LABORATORIES? Disruptions of normal sexual functions, such as the onset of puberty, menstrual bleeding, fertility, and of pregnancy, are sensitive indicators for a disruption in hormone secretion and function. Measuring hormones is often complicated and expensive. Still, for a number of diseases it is useful to measure sex hormones in order to connect the visible disruption unequivocally to a hormonal disruption. Measuring hormone levels is usually possible only in specialized laboratories.

Exact measurements are necessary, particularly if the problem is the treatment of sterility. In order to investigate for sterility in both men and women, experience and a detailed knowledge of the hormonal regulation system are necessary. Hormonal disruptions are only rarely the cause. It is possible, however, to induce pregnancy by hormone treatment. This discovery has made it possible, among other things, to perform in-vitro fertilization.

SUMMARY

Hormones affect our body in many different ways. This is particularly obvious with our sex hormones which cause gender differentiation between males and females. After birth the sex hormones estrogen and testosterone continue to play a part in the formation of our secondary sex characteristics, and in our reproductive ability. Specialized hormone laboratories can be asked to help in questions relating to sexual development, menstrual disorders, sterility, and the normal progress of a pregnancy.

APPENDIX: THE MOST SIGNIFICANT BLOOD VALUES

by G. Hoffman, MD
Adapted for N. America by Monique Jacques, MD

This final section provides a quick reference for those who are look-ing for concise information about frequently measured values in blood testing. But, for a better understanding of the measurements written in a lab report, you should, also read the chapters describing specific diseases.

We must also warn against over-interpreting a lab test result on the basis of these concise summaries. An accurate interpretation of laboratory values demands a great deal of experience, and in the end is always the responsibility of the physician who is treating you.

The normal ranges given here are based on the following text-books:

Textbook of Clinical Chemistry, ed. Norbert Tietz, W.B. Saun-ders, Philadelphia, PA, 1986.

Clinical Diagnosis and Management by Laboratory Methods, ed. John B. Henry, W.B. Saunders, Philadelphia, PA, 1991, in which an interested reader will find a wealth of further information.

As we have explained in detail earlier in this book, blood values outside the normal range should not necessarily be considered pathological, while, on the other hand, results inside the normal range cannot be a guarantee of health. Chapter 3 (From Blood Count to Diagnosis), in particular, provides information about the connections between blood values, their deviations from the normal range, and the illnesses that can be inferred from them.

What are considered normal ranges frequently differ even among laboratories, and we cannot, of course, include all the variations in this survey. This is particularly true for proteins, especially enzymes. Our ranges are based on the methods recommended in the texts listed above.

If there is any doubt, a particular normal range—if one is not printed on the laboratory report card—can be learned simply by asking the laboratory that conducted the test, or the patient's physician.

Under the heading *Units,* those that are commonly used in the U.S.A. are mentioned first. The other units are given beside these, and are sometimes supplemented by a figure in parentheses, which gives the conversion factors. It may be used to convert values from the first system of measurement into values for the second system, before the parentheses. To help explain this procedure, here is an example: Creatinine: mg/dl, mol/l (88.4) means that 1 mg/dl equals 88.4 mol/l.

General conversion factors within a single system of measurement, such as from milligrams (mg) into grams (g), and from deciliter (dl) into liter (l), can be found in the following chart.

►► *General Conversion Factors*

d = deci-   (tenths)
m = milli-   (thousandths)
μ = micro-   (millionths)
n = nano-   (billionths)
k = kilo-   (thousand)

UNIT OF MEASUREMENT	CONVERSION FACTOR
g–mg*	1,000
g–μg	1,000,000
mg–μg	1,000
mg–ng	1,000,000

mg–g	0.001
μg–g	0.000001
μg–mg	0.001
ng–mg	0.000001
l–dl	10
l–ml	1,000
dl–l	0.1
ml–l	0.001
g/dl–g/l	10
g/l–g/dl	0.1
U–mU	1,000
U–kU	0.001
mU–U	0.001
kU–U	1,000

*All conversion factors given for the gram system also apply to the mol system, for example mol to mmol: factor 1,000.

▸▸ *Alanine Aminotransferase*

Other names: Glutamate-pyruvate-transferase
Abbreviations: ALT, GPT, SGPT (serum GPT)
Description: Enzyme of the protein metabolism that is found primarily in the liver, and to a much lesser extent in skeletal and heart muscles. It enters the bloodstream following cell damage in these tissues.
Units: U/l, nkat/l
Normal range: Women and men: up to 55 U/l. Children have a somewhat higher normal value.
Medical significance: ALT (GPT) is used mainly to detect diseases of the liver. Extremely elevated levels (50 to 100 times normal) are found in hepatocellular disease, liver infections (hepatitis), and disruptions of blood supply to the liver. In diseases of the heart and the muscles, this enzyme is often measured in order to better judge the tissue origin of elevated levels of other enzymes (creatinekinase, aspartate aminotransferase, lactate-dehydrogenase).

▸▸ *Albumin*

Description: By weight, albumin is the most important protein in our serum. It is synthesized in the liver mainly from food proteins.

Units (factor): g/l, g/dl, mmol/l (0.0152)
Normal range: 36–52 g/l
Medical significance: Albumin is useful in estimating roughly how much protein is being synthesized by the liver. Lower levels are due to decreased liver performance, long term protein deficiencies as in malnutrition, or protein loss at a higher rate than the liver can compensate for, as in kidney disease or intestinal disease. True increases in albumin blood levels almost never occur; elevated levels are mostly due to dehydration.

►► *Alcohol*

Other names: Ethyl alcohol, Ethanol, C_2H_5OH
Description: Alcohol is usually consumed in beverages, or, more rarely, is infused. It is metabolized in the liver into acetate (acetaldehyde and acetic acid).
Units (factor): mg/dl, mmol/l (0.217)
Normal range: Without ingestion alcohol is not measurable in the blood. The limit from which the presence of alcohol can be detected with certainty depends on the test method. Since blood cells contain less alcohol than serum following consumption, alcohol concentrations are about 20 percent lower in whole blood than in centrifuged serum or plasma. Legal limits for driving are given for total blood alcohol rather than serum or plasma alcohol. In order to be legally significant, alcohol levels must be measured at a certified institute such as a hospital.
Medical significance: In high concentrations, alcohol can cause decreased inhibition, incoordination, stupor, coma, seizures, and death. Chronic abuse causes stomach and liver damage. Changes in behavior depend mainly on levels of tolerance, but usually begin to occur at blood concentrations of 75 to 150 mg/dl. Slight, moderate, and severe states of intoxication occur at levels of 150 to 250 mg/dl. Loss of consciousness and a possibly fatal coma due to breathing paralysis occur at levels of 300 to 500 mg/dl.

►► *Alkaline Phosphatase*

Abbreviation: AP, ALK.phos
Description: AP is an enzyme that is present in the liver, and also in bones, intestine, kidneys, and the placenta. The name alkaline phos-

phatase covers an entire family of different enzymes with some disparate qualities. They can be distinguished further with the help of an isoenzyme test.

Units: U/l

Normal range: Females 1–15 years: < 350 U/l; over 15 years: 25–100 U/l. Males 1–12 years: < 350 U/l; 12–15 years: < 500 U/l; over 20 years: 25–100 U/l. Values for children during growth phases are significantly higher than adult values due to an AP isoenzyme released by the bones. AP is also elevated during pregnancy (to a maximum of approximately twice normal).

Medical significance: AP is mainly used to detect diseases of the liver, the bile ducts, and the bones. Particularly high values (about 5 to 10 times normal) are seen during disorders in which bile flow is obstructed, such as a blockage of the bile flow due to gallstones. Often in these cases icterus also occurs. Bone diseases like osteoporosis usually cause no or only slight elevation in AP levels. Isoenzyme tests may be useful in such cases. Some bone disorders, such as Paget's disease, may cause moderate increases in alkaline phosphatase.

▶▶ *Alpha-Fetoprotein*

Abbreviation: AFP

Description: AFP is a protein of the group of alpha-globulins, which is produced by the yolk sac and fetal liver. In adults it plays no significant role.

Units: ng/ml, mg/dl

Normal range: Up to 20 ng/ml. At 16 weeks' gestation, AFP levels in fetal serum are elevated to about 100 mg/l (5,000 times adult levels), but after the first year children have about the same values as adults. During pregnancy, AFP increases to a maximum of about 50 times normal (32nd to 36th week of pregnancy) and then drops again to normal.

Medical significance: Slight to moderate increases in level (up to about 50 times normal) occur with various liver diseases (hepatitis, alcoholism, cirrhosis). Values that are up to 1,000 times normal indicate tumors originating in liver, testes, or ovaries. AFP is therefore considered to be a tumor marker. It can be used to evaluate therapeutic measures and the progress of these tumors.

▸▸ *Amylase*

Other names: Alpha-amylase

Description: Amylase is an enzyme from the pancreas and other salivary glands which can also, if rarely and in small amounts, be formed in other organs (lungs, intestines, ovaries). It is used to digest starch. The name amylase covers two different enzymes which are called p– and s–amylase (p for pancreas, s for salivary gland), and which can be distinguished from each other with a special isoenzyme test.

Units: U/l

Normal range: Differs depending on test used.

Medical significance: Amylase levels are elevated, especially during diseases of the pancreas, although the amount of increase is not indicative of the severity of the disease. A three-fold or greater elevation is usually due to acute inflammation of the pancreas. Medically less significant and sometimes even misleading elevations are found in association with kidney disease, mumps, and abdominal pregnancy, and macroamylasemia. Some of these increases may be resolved if, instead of total amylase, only p–amylase is measured with the help of an isoenzyme test.

▸▸ *APO A–I, APO A–II, APO B*—See Lipoproteins

▸▸ *Aspartate Aminotransferase*

Other names: Glutamate-oxalacetate-transaminase

Abbreviations: AST, SGOT (serum GOT)

Description: AST (SGOT) is an enzyme of our protein metabolism which is present mainly in the liver, but is also found in skeletal and heart muscle, as well as within red blood corpuscles (erythrocytes). Following damage to any of these cell types it is released into the bloodstream.

Units: U/l

Normal range: Women and men: up to 50 U/l. Children have somewhat higher normal ranges.

Medical significance: It is used mainly in detecting liver diseases and in monitoring therapeutic progress following heart and skeletal muscle damage. Very high levels (50 to 100 times normal) occur most commonly during infectious liver disease (hepatitis) and circulatory disturbances involving the liver. Falsely elevated values occur if erythrocytes disintegrate prior to analyzing the blood sample.

▶▶ *Bilirubin*

Abbreviation: TBIL (total bilirubin)
Description: Bilirubin is yellow in color, and is a catabolic product of red blood cell pigment. (See Hemoglobin, below.) It is altered in the liver, and is partially excreted in the bile into the intestine. It may also pass through the kidneys into the urine. The brown and yellow coloring of stool and urine is mainly due to hemoglobin catabolic products, such as bilirubin and related substances. In our blood, the different forms of bilirubin are known as direct and indirect bilirubin. The sum total of all bilirubin is referred to as total bilirubin (TBIL).
Units (factor): mg/dl, μmol/l. (17.1)
Normal range: Up to 1.2 mg/dl. Newborns have a level ten times higher than adults. This normalizes during the first few weeks.
Medical significance: Moderately elevated blood levels of bilirubin may be recognized by a yellow tint of the skin and/or the eyes (jaundice, or in Latin, *icterus*). It occurs with inflammation of the liver (hepatitis), obstruction of bile ducts (as with gallstones), or, more rarely, with pancreatic disease or during increased red blood cell destruction. In premature infants without a fully functional liver, bilirubin levels may be increased. Persistently elevated bilirubin levels may also be seen in infants who suffer a maternal immune reaction against their red blood cells (hemolytic disease of the newborn due to Rh incompatibility). A high proportion of indirect bilirubin suggests a disease of the liver or increased red blood cell destruction.

▶▶ *Blood Group Factors*

Description: Blood groups are genetically transmitted characteristics of red blood cells that are, among other things, responsible for compatibility with donor blood. Most of the blood group factors are proteins that contain different amounts of carbohydrates, and occur on the surface of our blood cells. The most important ones are designated by letters (A, B, C (c), D (d), and E (e). If neither A nor B are present, we speak of blood group "O". The factors C, D, and E are also called rhesus factors (Rh).
Medical significance: Transfusions of donor blood belonging to incompatible blood types causes defensive reactions of our immune system that include dizziness, shivering, loss of consciousness, kidney failure, and death due to shock. Before each transfusion the blood group of the donor and recipient must be identified and tested for

compatibility by mixing both types of blood in a test tube. This is known as cross matching.

▶▶ *Blood Sedimentation*

Other names: Erythrocyte sedimentation rate
Abbreviation: ESR
Description: The erythrocyte sedimentation rate, according to the Westergren method, expresses the distance in millimeters by which blood cells descend within one hour in a thin, standardized glass tube. The sedimentation rate is influenced by the red blood cells' size, shape, and natural electrical charge, as well as by the composition of the plasma and various other, still unknown factors.
Units: mm/hour
Normal range: Females under 50 years: up to 20 mm/hr; males under 50 years: up to 15 mm/hr.
Medical significance: Values above 25 mm/hour in men less than 85 years or women less than 50 years suggest a defensive reaction within the body (such as a bacterial infection, an inflammatory process, tumors, or rheumatoid arthritis). Elevated levels may also be seen during a normal pregnancy. Significantly decreased values, around 1 mm/hour, can be seen during some viral infections due to changes in erythrocyte shape, for example, sickle cell anemia, increased erythrocyte number (erythrocytosis), and congestive heart failure.

▶▶ *Blood Sugar*—See Glucose

▶▶ *Calcium*

Abbreviation: Ca
Description: Calcium is one of the most important minerals in our body. It is of central importance to bone strength, and it regulates numerous metabolic processes. Keeping the calcium concentration in our blood and cells constant is the function of a very complicated regulatory mechanism in which, among other substances, parathormon from the parathyroid gland and Vitamin D play an important role. About half of all calcium in the blood is bound to proteins, mainly albumin. The free (unbound) portion of the calcium, however, is responsible for calcium's biological effects.

Units (factor): mg/dl, mmol/l (0.2495)

Normal range: 9.2–11 mg/dl (2.3–2.74 mmol/l)

Medical significance: Variations in calcium concentration can be caused by disruptions in the sensitive regulatory mechanism, or by changes in the binding proteins. In the first case, severe complaints may be expected. Calcium deficiencies lead to muscle spasms and shaking (tetany), as well as a gradual decalcification of the bones. Excessively high calcium levels cause patients to experience such symptoms as nausea and muscular weakness. If, on the other hand, a depressed calcium level is the result of a decrease in binding proteins, these symptoms do not appear, since only the bound—the biologically inert—calcium portion has been affected.

▶▶ *Carcinoembryonal Antigen*

Abbreviation: CEA

Description: CEA is a carbohydrate containing protein whose function is still unknown. It is formed in various cells (lungs, spleen, blood cells) and metabolized in the liver. In healthy people it is present only in trace amounts.

Units: ng/ml

Normal range: Differs depending on test method (up to a maximum of 10 ng/ml).

Medical significance: Slight to moderate increases (two- to four-fold) are found in heavy smokers and in diseases affecting the liver, lungs, intestines, and pancreas. Higher values suggest a tumor of these organs, of the female breast, or reproductive organs (ovaries, uterus). That is why CEA is included among tumor markers. It is useful for therapeutic monitoring but not in searching for a tumor.

▶▶ *Chloride*

Abbreviation: Cl

Description: By amount, chloride is the most important negatively charged blood ion. It is also a part of table salt (sodium chloride, or NaCl) and hydrochloric acid (HCl).

Units: mmol/l

Normal range: 98–106 mmol/l

Medical significance: Depressed levels occur mainly after loss due to vomiting (stomach acid) and excessive doses of certain medications that increase urine secretion (salt loss). Elevated levels occur with severe diarrhea. A number of rare diseases of the endocrine glands lead to elevated or depressed chloride values.

►► *Cholesterol*

Description: Cholesterol is a metabolic product belonging to the lipids (fats). It is a component of cell membranes, and is an important initial substance in the hormone synthesis of sex hormones. In the blood it occurs in a "packaged" form as lipoprotein. Depending on the different forms of lipoprotein, a distinction is made between HDL-cholesterol and LDL-cholesterol, as well as a few other cholesterol subgroups.

Units (factor): mg/dl, mmol/l (0.0259)

Normal range: The normal range for cholesterol depends largely on the diet of a given population. For example, in Europe the lower level of the range is about 150 mg/dl, with an upper limit of 200 mg/dl + years of age in mg/dl. In the U.S.A. the upper limit is considered to be 220 mg/dl.

Because of wide fluctuations, the normal range for cholesterol is of limited medical significance. More interesting is the ideal range which, experts agree, should be less than 200 mg/dl and which is connected with a particularly low risk of heart attack, as seen in Chinese people. However, the different effects of HDL- and LDL-cholesterol must be considered when comparing test results to ideal ranges. The information can be misleading if only the total mg/dl is read. (See Lipoproteins, below, for further discussion.)

Medical significance: Depressed levels can be found in cases of extreme malnutrition, and thyroid hyperfunction. Elevated levels are only due in part to excessive supply. Genetic factors, for example, the number of LDL-receptors on the body's cells, seem to be more important. Elevated cholesterol values are also associated with thyroid hypofunction, diabetes mellitus, and other metabolic disorders.

The importance of cholesterol levels in preventive medicine is based on the relationship between elevated cholesterol and increased risk of heart attack. This relationship is significant only for the LDL portion of cholesterol, and for some other cholesterol subgroups (Lp–a), but not for HDL-cholesterol, which is its second most common form. (See Lipoproteins, below.)

▸▸ *Cortisol*

Description: Cortisol is a hormone formed from cholesterol and secreted by the adrenal cortex. It has a number of different effects on our metabolism. For example, it increases blood sugar, and it retards inflammatory reactions. Cortisol secretion is increased in response to stress, such as surgery, infection, or hemorrhage.
Units (factor): μg/dl, mmol/l (27.59)
Normal range: At 8 A.M., 5–23 μg/dl. At midnight, 0–5 μg/dl. During the day, levels tend to fall, but may increase in response to stress.
Medical significance: Cortisol acts as a damper for numerous symptoms of inflammatory disorders, such as swelling and pain. It is therefore used in many forms of medication. Pathologically elevated levels at which the typical daily rhythm is disrupted are most likely due to an adrenal gland tumor, a pituitary tumor, or a tumor in another site, such as the lungs. Depressed levels, on the other hand, are found when the adrenal glands or pituitary are not functioning.

▸▸ *Creatinekinase*

Other names: Creatinephosphokinase (outdated)
Abbreviations: CK, (CPK)
Description: CK is an enzyme that is responsible for energy production in the muscles. It occurs in skeletal muscles, in the heart, and in the brain. There are a total of three CK isoenzymes: CK–MM (M for muscle), CK–BB (B for brain), and CK–MB (a mixed form of muscle and brain enzyme), which is found mainly in the heart muscle. Most of the CK in our blood belongs to the MM type.
Units: U/l
Normal range: 30–70 U/l, newborns 3x adult values
Medical significance: Increased CK activity in the blood suggests muscle damage. The spectrum of possible causes ranges from sore muscles to infarct. A more sensitive diagnostic tool is the measurement of CK isoenzyme activity. Falsely elevated levels appear after muscle injections and as the result of a harmless CK variant (Macro–CK–BB).

►► *Creatinine*

Description: Creatinine is a product of the muscles' metabolism. It is secreted by the kidneys.
Units (factor): mg/dl, μmol/l (88.4)
Normal range: Varies according to test method. Normal range: 0.5–1.2 mg/dl.
Medical significance: Elevated levels suggest reduced kidney function, but are also common in body-builders and athletes with a large muscle mass. In order to detect even minor kidney damage it is common to measure creatinine in both blood and urine over the course of an entire day, and then to compute the creatinine clearance as a measure of kidney performance. It indicates the kidney's filtration performance, in clearing creatinine from the blood, in ml/min (normally up to 139 ml/min).

►► *Erythrocytes*

Other names: Red blood corpuscles, red blood cells
Abbreviation: RBC
Description: Erythrocytes are formed in the bone marrow and live about 120 days, during which time they circulate in the bloodstream. Their task is to transport oxygen from the lungs to the organs. The blood's red color is due to hemoglobin, the iron-containing, oxygen-binding protein in the erythrocytes.
Units: number per microliter
Normal range: Females: 4.2–5.4 million per microliter, Males: 4.6–6.2 million per microliter. Newborns have slightly higher values.
Medical significance: The number of erythrocytes is determined by their rate of formation in the bone marrow, and the rate of destruction or loss due to bleeding. Changes in the body's fluid balance, like dehydration, also lead to changes in the number of erythrocytes per microliter of blood. Decreased levels are found most often in cases of iron deficiency, blood loss, as well as Vitamin B12 deficiency, or, more rarely, due to hemolysis and some congenital diseases. Increases are rare and are usually due to concentration of the RBC's, as in dehydration. Only in a rare disease, polycythemia vera, does the formation rate in the bone marrow increase. Microscopic examination of the erythrocytes includes an examination of their shape, which provides information about genetic variations in RBC formation, and damage due to other causes.

▸▸ *Ferritin*

Description: Ferritin is an important iron-binding substance which is found in numerous cells. Most of it is found in the liver, where iron from the food is stored for blood formation and other metabolic processes. Ferritin that is measurable in the blood reflects the body's reserves of iron.

Units: ng/ml, μg/l

Normal range: Depends very much on measuring technique. Women are usually measured at 12–150 ng/ml, men at 15–200 ng/ml. Children and seniors can have even higher values.

Medical significance: Elevated ferritin levels often indicate liver disease, an inflammatory process, or possibly a cancer, or, more rarely still, excessive iron absorption. Depressed levels occur with iron deficiencies and other forms of blood loss, usually of a chronic nature.

▸▸ *Gamma Glutamyl Transferase*

Abbreviation: GGT

Description: Gamma-GT is an enzyme of the liver and kidneys. However, we measure only the liver enzyme, which plays an important role in protein metabolism. The kidney enzyme does not enter the blood and is secreted into the urine.

Units: U/l

Normal range: Females and males 1–30 years: to 60 U/l. Newborns and infants can have values up to 100 U/l.

Medical significance: Depressed levels are of no medical significance. Increased enzyme activity suggests damage to the liver or the bile ducts which is most often caused by alcohol, medication, or chronic obstruction to bile flow. GGT may be elevated in alcoholics even without liver disease. Other causes for an increase are inflammation and tumors of the liver or bile ducts, as well as gallstones.

▸▸ *Glucose*

Other names: Blood sugar

Description: Glucose is the most important sugar in the body. It is absorbed from food and is used by all cells as a source of energy. Some types of cells, in particular red blood cells, are dependent on glucose as an energy source because they are not able to metabolize fat. Because of its great importance, our body uses hormones to keep the glucose level as constant as possible. In many countries blood sugar measurement is the most common blood test. It is usually conducted from serum, but rarely also from whole blood, where levels are somewhat lower.

Units (factor): mg/dl, mmol/l (0.0556)

Normal range (serum): fasting level: up to 140 mg/dl. 30 to 60 minutes after a meal: increases to approximately 10–15 mg/dl over fasting level (post-prandial blood sugar).

Medical significance: Significantly elevated blood sugar levels suggest diabetes mellitus, or very rarely, other disruptions in glucose metabolism (for example, overproduction of cortisol in the adrenal glands). There are, however, transitional states between the normal level and one that signifies diabetes, and these can be determined by blood sugar measurements following standardized patient preparation.

For this purpose the patient, who has been instructed to eat carbohydrate-rich food the day before the examination, is given a glucose solution that is soon absorbed into the bloodstream. The blood sugar level is measured just prior to this glucose tolerance test, and then repeat measurements are taken every 30 to 60 minutes. From the initial increase and subsequent drop in levels we can assess metabolic performance.

Criteria differ somewhat among countries. As a general rule, values of more than 200 mg/dl in serum are consistent with diabetes.

Slightly elevated levels are found in latent diabetes mellitus, but may also be seen post-operatively, in the presence of pancreatic disease, during periods of stress, or with use of certain medications, like oral contraceptives.

▸▸ *Glutamate-Oxalacetate-Transaminase* (GOT)
—See Aspartate Aminotransferase

▸▸ *Glutamate-Pyruvate-Transferase* (GPT)—See Alanine Aminotransferase

▸▸ HDL-*Cholesterol*—See Cholesterol and Lipoproteins

►► *Hematocrit*

Abbreviation: Hct
Description: The hematocrit is a blood measurement that indicates the proportional volume in percent of red blood cells in the blood.
Units: percent
Normal range: Females: 38% to 47%; males: 40% to 54%
Medical significance: The hematocrit provides information about the red blood corpuscles, which are important in supplying oxygen to the body. At the same time the hematocrit measurement indicates the blood's liquid proportion (plasma), as the remaining percentage of a total of 100 percent. Depressed hematocrit levels indicate anemia or an excess of liquid in the blood, while elevated levels indicate an increase in the number of erythrocytes or a decrease in blood liquid. If the hematocrit value is divided by the number of erythrocytes, the resulting term expresses the volume of these cells as mean corpuscular volume (MCV).

►► *Hemoglobin*

Abbreviation: Hb
Description: Hemoglobin is an iron-containing protein in the erythrocytes which is responsible for the blood's red color. It binds oxygen that enters the body through the lungs, and transports it to the various organs.
Units: g/dl, g/l
Normal range: Females: 12–16 g/dl; males: 13.5–18 g/dl
Medical significance: The measurement of hemoglobin, concentration, besides the erythrocyte count and hematocrit, is used to diagnose anemia, or an increase in the number of blood cells. A decrease in hemoglobin is referred to as anemia. Anemia has many causes, which include disruption of blood formation in the bone marrow due to iron deficiency, porphyria, or genetically based hemoglobin variations. Blood loss during menstruation or due to hemorrhage may also cause a decrease in Hb. An increase in hemoglobin occurs with dwelling at high altitudes, athletic training, and increased formation of red blood corpuscles in the bone marrow (polycythemia).

Of medical significance is a special subgroup of hemoglobin, referred to as hemoglobin A_{1C} (abbreviated as Hb A_{1C}). It is formed from hemoglobin and blood sugar, and is increased in diabetics as a result of elevated blood sugar levels. By testing Hb A_{1C} levels, the physician can determine whether or not medication levels for diabetes are optimal.

▶▶ *Hydroxybutyrate-Dehydrogenase*—See Lactate-dehydrogenase

▶▶ *Immune Globulins*

Other names: Gamma-globulins, antibodies
Abbreviations: IgA, IgE, IgG, IgM, IgD (see below)
Description: Immune globulins are proteins which are formed by special defensive cells (lymphocytes, plasma cells). They are formed in response to and interact with foreign substances. In our blood, immune globulins are present in a number of different classes that are designated by the letters A, E, G, and M—hence immune globulin A, which is abbreviated IgA. Each class contains thousands of individual antibodies against a wide variety of substances and organisms.

The four globulin classes have somewhat different functions. IgM takes part, among other functions, in the early defense against infections, while IgG is formed at a later stage, but in greater amounts. IgA is the immune globulin of mucous membranes, and IgE is formed in response to large intruding organisms, especially worms, and in allergies. A fifth immune globulin, IgD is found in the blood only in trace amounts and is therefore rarely measured.
Units: g/l, mg/dl
Normal range: IgG 8–18 g/l, IgA 1.1–5.6 g/l, IgM 0.5–2.2 g/l, IgE up to 0.4 mg/l. As a rule, children have lower immune globulin levels than adults. Only IgG tends to be higher during childhood and adolescence.
Medical significance: Immune globulin concentrations in the blood are closely connected to our defense system's performance. During most infectious diseases the formation of immune globulins is increased. However, this increase does not always lead to an increase in values beyond the normal range. This is due to the fact that only individual forms of antibodies are being produced in large amounts. Elevated total values are usually due to chronic liver disease. Low immune globulin values may indicate a reduced defensive ability.

In rare cases, and mainly in older people, an increase in a "clone" of immune globulin producing cells in the bone marrow can take place. This is known as monoclonal gammopathy. In these cases the affected immune globulin class has extremely high values. Extreme elevation of monoclonal immune globulin occur in a cancer known as multiple myeloma.

►► Iron

Abbreviation: Fe
Description: Iron is a mineral which occurs in blood only in trace amounts. Most of it is bound to the proteins ferritin and transferrin. Its main function is to bind oxygen in the red blood pigment, hemoglobin. It is also a component of various enzymes, particularly within macrophages, which are responsible for defending against foreign bodies, for disposal of dead cell material, and for destroying tumors.
Units (factor): μg/dl, μmol/l, (0.1791)
Normal range: Fluctuates widely depending on age and gender. In women of reproductive age, about 30–150 μg/dl, somewhat higher in men and children. The lower value in women is due to loss during menstruation, pregnancy, and lactation.
Medical significance: Iron deficiencies are most commonly triggered by dietary deficiencies or bleeding. In association with inflammation and malignant tumors, iron levels may be low. Depressed levels are often accompanied by fatigue and pallor. Deficiencies may also be due to a disruption in the intestine's ability to absorb iron. Increased concentrations are rare and occur in certain diseases in the blood and liver. In order to determine the exact reasons for a change in iron level, it is usually necessary to conduct further testing, such as measuring ferritin and transferrin, and calculating the blood's iron-binding capacity (known as TIBC, the total iron-binding capacity).

►► Lactate-Dehydrogenase

Abbreviations: LDH, LD
Description: LDH is an enzyme involved in sugar metabolism, and is found in all of our body's cells, but in particularly high concentrations in the liver, muscles, and erythrocytes. There are altogether five different isoenzymes which are referred to as LD–1 through LD–5. These isoenzymes appear in different organs in different concentrations. For example, LD–1 is seen in greatest concentrations in heart

muscle and erythrocytes, while LD–5 activity is greatest in the liver.
Units: U/l
Normal range: 45–100 U/l. Children to 250 U/l. Newborns to 450 U/l.
Medical significance: As LDH is present in large amounts in nearly all cells, its appearance in the blood is a good indicator that there is cell damage somewhere in the body. However, increased LDH levels do not provide specific information about their organ of origin. A certain differentiation is possible due to the identification of isoenzymes, but more commonly transaminase and creatinekinase are measured to distinguish between liver and muscle cell damage. Very high LDH values (around 1,000 U/l) appear not only in cases of liver or muscle damage, but also when erythrocytes are destroyed (hemolysis). After heart attacks, LDH increases significantly after a few days, and then slowly drops to normal levels again, so that infarctions can be recognized even after a week has passed.

Falsely elevated LDH levels appear when erythrocytes are destroyed while the blood sample is being drawn or transported to the lab.

▶▶ LDL-*Cholesterol*—See Cholesterol and Lipoproteins

▶▶ *Leukocytes*

Other names: White blood corpuscles, white cells
Abbreviation: WBC (white blood cells)
Description: Leukocytes are a group of blood cells containing a nucleus, that are formed in the bone marrow. Their primary task is to defend the body against foreign substances and microorganisms, but they also destroy dead cells and malignant cells. Leukocytes are subdivided into granulocytes (about 60 percent), monocytes (about 5 percent), and lymphocytes (about 35 percent), and other, smaller subgroups.
Units: number of cells per μl
Normal range: 4,300 to 10,000 per μl. Newborns and children can have higher values (up to 30,000 in newborns).
Medical significance: An increase in leukocytes can be seen during many inflammatory reactions. Slight increases can be seen during mild to moderate infections, after physical exertion, and even after meals. Two and three times normal values are found during more se-

vere diseases. Extremely high numbers (100,000 per μl and more) suggest malignant leukocyte formation in the bone marrow (leukemia). Decreased numbers of leukocytes can be observed during some infectious diseases (for example typhoid and viral flu), in those whose immune system has been compromised (for example, by radiation therapy), and in AIDS patients, as well as during rare allergic reactions to painkillers and antibiotics.

▶▶ *Lipase*

Description: Lipase is similar to p—amylase in that it is a digestive enzyme from the pancreas. It is secreted into the intestine following the consumption of food, and breaks up fats. It is excreted mainly through the intestine. The lipase that can be detected in the blood is mainly excreted through the kidneys.

Units: U/l

Normal range: Depending on method usually up to 280 U/l

Medical significance: Increased levels of lipase are most commonly used in the diagnosis of acute pancreatitis.

▶▶ *Lipoproteins*

Description: Lipoproteins are a mixture of fats (lipids) and proteins. These proteins are referred to as apoproteins, and serve as carriers for the blood fats they contain. Lipoproteins are a mixture of substances, most of which can be measured individually. The most frequently measured apoproteins are Apo A–I, Apo A–II, and Apo B. Cholesterol, the most important fat component of lipoproteins, is also measured.

There are three main categories of lipoproteins: "high density" lipoproteins (abbreviated HDL), "low density" lipoproteins (abbreviated LDL), and the "very low density" lipoproteins (abbreviated VLDL). Of these, usually the cholesterol portion is measured, and is then called HDL-, LDL-, or VLDL-cholesterol.

Other lipoproteins that are occasionally measured are lipoprotein X, and lipoprotein (a).

Units: mg/dl, μmol/l

Reference interval (normal range): Lipoproteins and their components are judged partly according to normal ranges and partly by ideal ranges. As a rule, elevated levels are considered unfavorable. Exceptions are HDL-cholesterol, Apo A–I and Apo A–II, in which elevated values mean protection against arteriosclerosis. For all three substances, the reference interval for women of reproductive age is about 10 mg/dl higher than the following values.

HDL-cholesterol: 35–55 mg/dl

LDL-cholesterol: up to 150 mg/dl

VLDL-cholesterol: up to 35 mg/dl

Apo A–I: 90–130 mg/dl

Apo A–II: 30–50 mg/dl

Apo B: about 65–120 mg/dl

Lipoprotein (a): depending on method, up to about 50 mg/dl

Medical significance: Lipoproteins play an important role in the development of arteriosclerosis and its consequences, in particular heart attacks (infarctions). As a simplified rule we can say that high LDL and low HDL values increase the risk of infarction, while high HDL and low LDL values help decrease it. Endurance athletes and chronic alcoholics have a favorable ratio of HDL and LDL. Women also tend to have higher HDL-cholesterol levels than men. This advantage disappears after menopause, or if oral contraceptives are used. Unfavorable ratios are often found in smokers and in people with sedentary lifestyles.

Apo A–I and Apo A–II can be considered as similiar to HDL, and Apo B as similiar to LDL-cholesterol. Increased concentrations of lipoprotein (a) favor the development of arteriosclerosis. Lipoprotein X does not appear in the blood of healthy people, and is not involved in the development of arteriosclerosis. When it appears, it points to a disease of the bile ducts.

▸▸ *Magnesium*

Abbreviation: Mg

Description: Magnesium, like sodium, potassium, and calcium, is a mineral substance in our blood that fulfills numerous metabolic tasks in the cells. It is especially important for the energy metabolism in our organs and the excitability of muscles and nerves. It is consumed in food and secreted in urine and stool.

Units (factor): mg/dl, mEq/l, mmol/l (mg/dl to mmol/l, 0.4113; mEq/l to mmol/l, 0.5)

Normal range: 1.8–3 mg/dl or 1.3–2.1 mEq/l (0.7–1 mmol/l). Somewhat higher in infants.

Medical significance: Since by far the largest share of our magnesium reserves is kept within the cells, magnesium concentrations in the blood can provide only incomplete information about the actual supply in the body. Mild magnesium deficiencies are accompanied by fatigue and weakness, in severe cases by muscle cramps, seizures, and heart rhythm disruptions. The causes are low levels of magnesium in the diet, for example, from alcoholism, diseases of the digestive organs, and in rare cases, medications that affect the kidneys. Extremely high levels, on the other hand, occur almost always due to severe kidney dysfunction.

▸▸ Partial Thromboplastin Time

Abbreviations: PTT, a-PTT (activated PTT)
Description: PTT is a measuring technique which provides information about the entire coagulation system's function.
Units: seconds (sec.)
Normal range: depending on method, 25–35 seconds.
Medical significance: An increased PTT suggests a disruption in coagulation performance and an increase in clotting time. This disruption may be congenital (as in hemophiliacs), or may appear as the result of another disease process, such as liver disease. Most frequently, however, the physician causes an increase in PTT time by medication that is designed to counteract tendencies toward thrombosis. In particular, the effects of the anticoagulant drug Heparin are monitored by means of the PTT.

▸▸ Potassium

Abbreviation: K
Description: Potassium is, after sodium, the second most important positively charged blood mineral. Within our cells it is the most prevalent among mineral ions. It is absorbed from food, and is responsible for many different metabolic processes, as well as the electrical excitability of nerve and muscle cells. It is secreted through the intestine and the kidneys, and also in perspiration.
Units: mmol/l, mEq/l
Normal range: 3.8–5 mmol/l. Somewhat higher (up to about 6 mmol/l) in newborns and infants.
Medical significance: Since potassium is of the greatest importance for regulation of nearly all vital processes, our body keeps the concentration of potassium in the blood and in the cells extraordinarily constant. Fluctuations both upward and downward are seen during kidney diseases, and as a result of medications which stimulate urination.

Decreased levels also occur with diarrhea, vomiting, overdoses of laxatives, and some rare diseases of the adrenal glands. The greatest danger that results from a disruption in potassium levels is a change in the heart muscle's excitability, leading to disruptions in heart function.

►► Prostatic Acid Phosphatase

Abbreviation: PAP
Description: The group of acid phosphatase enzymes, like alkaline phosphatase, constitute a family of isoenzymes. They appear in various distribution patterns in the prostate, bones, liver, and in the blood cells.

Usually only the prostate isoenzyme is measured. Women have measurable amounts of total acid phosphatase but not prostatic acid phosphatase. A diagnostic improvement has been achieved recently by the discovery and measurement of prostate-specific antigen (PSA), which occurs mostly in the prostate and is not identical with prostatic acid phosphatase.
Units: U/l, μg/l (Direct conversion not possible.)
Normal range: Depending on technique, usually around 2 U/l or μg/l.
Medical significance: An increase in prostate-specific enzyme indicates a tumor, either benign or malignant, of the male prostate gland. The higher the measurement, the more likely a malignancy is present which has spread outside the prostate gland. A manual examination by the physician can also lead to elevated levels, which is why this test must always be conducted before the manual examination.

►► Protein

Other names: Total protein
Abbreviation: TP
Description: Proteins are the largest and most varied class of substances in our blood. They include transport proteins like albumin and transferase, enzymes such as creatinekinase and amylase, defensive proteins such as antibodies and C–reactive protein, hormones, and many more.
Units: g/dl, g/l
Normal range: 6–7.8 g/dl in serum. Less in newborns.
Medical significance: Measuring total blood protein is a quick indicator of a person's general state of health. Divergences from the normal

range can point to changes in individual proteins (especially albumin and defensive proteins), or they can be caused by changes in fluid levels in our body. Increased concentrations are seen with dehydration, while decreased concentrations may be due to insufficient heart function. In all of these cases further testing, (for example, measuring albumin or protein electrophoresis), will be necessary.

▸▸ *Protein Electrophoresis*

Description: Electrophoresis is a special analysis technique which is used to separate blood proteins into individual subgroups, or fractions, in order to facilitate their further analysis. Normally five fractions are obtained, which are referred to as the albumin fraction, alpha–1, alpha–2, beta, and gamma globulin fraction.
Units: percent (of the five fractions)
Medical significance: Electrophoretic percentages have no particular medical significance. More important is their distribution pattern, which is plotted as a curve containing five "hills" and "valleys." It allows the physician to diagnose acute and chronic response to stress, as well as diseases of the liver, kidneys, and plasma cells.

▸▸ *Reticulocytes*

Abbreviation: Retics
Description: Reticulocytes are immature progenitors of the erythrocytes—the red blood corpuscles. They are formed in the bone marrow during RBC formation and, in healthy people, are released into the bloodstream in small amounts, together with mature erythrocytes.
Units: Number per µl, percentage of mature erythrocytes.
Normal range: 25,000–75,000 per µl blood, or 0.5%–1.5 percent (men: 1%–2.5 percent) of erythrocytes.
Medical significance: An increase in the number of reticulocytes suggests an accelerated rate of RBC formation in the bone marrow. This is the case mainly after blood loss, or destruction of the blood cells (hemolysis). The number of reticulocytes also increases during treatment for anemia, for example, with iron supplements, as a sign of therapeutic success. Decreased counts signal a disruption in new RBC formation, which may be due to kidney failure, radiation, or to medication which inhibits cell formation (cytostatica).

▸▸ *Sodium*

Other names: Natrium (Latin), salt
Abbreviation: Na
Description: By volume, sodium is the most important mineral substance in our blood, and a component of table salt (NaCl). It is absorbed from food and excreted by the kidneys. Its main function is to maintain the electrical charge of cell membranes in our body. It is usually measured along with potassium.
Units: mmol/l, mEq/l
Normal range: 136–142 mmol/l
Medical significance: A constant concentration of sodium in our blood is of such vital importance that deviations from the normal level are fairly rare. Most commonly they occur in connection with heart and kidney insufficiencies. Other causes for changes in sodium levels are diseases of the hormone-producing adrenal glands or the neuro-hypophysis. Medication can also affect the sodium balance.

▸▸ *Thrombocytes*

Other names: Platelets
Abbreviation: plts
Description: Thrombocytes are cell fractions without nuclei that are formed in the bone marrow. During coagulation they clump together in a platelet thrombus, and in this way help to quickly seal wounds.
Units: Number per μl
Normal range: 150,000 to 450,000 per μl
Medical significance: A decrease in the number of platelets may be a sign of increased coagulation activity due to severe injuries, inflammation, or surgical operations (disseminated intravascular coagulation). Other possible causes include insufficient formation in the bone marrow, due to infection, malignancy, radiation, or a reaction to certain medications. Increased values indicate an increased coagulatory readiness which occurs with various inflammatory disorders, disorders of bone marrow proliferation, malignancy, or reactive processes. The thrombocyte count can also be temporarily increased following the surgical removal of the spleen.

►► *Thyrotropic Hormone*

Other names: Thyrotropin
Abbreviation: TSH
Description: TSH is formed in the anterior pituitary gland, and stimulates the thyroid gland to produce hormones.
Units: μIU/ml, μg/dl
Normal range: 0.5–5 μIU/ml. In newborns, up to 23 ng/dl.
Medical significance: TSH concentration in the blood provides information about the thyroid gland's performance. Normally, if its activity is too low, the hypophysis increases TSH production. On the other hand, if it is too high, TSH production is decreased. A very low TSH value may indicate a thyroid hyperfunction (hyperthyroidism), and a strongly increased value indicates a thyroid hypofunction (hypothyroidism).

The early recognition of elevated TSH concentrations is particularly important in newborns suffering from congenital hypothyroidism, since, if this disease is not treated in time, it can lead to severe mental retardation and physical abnormalities. In patients suffering from goiter (an enlargement of the thyroid gland), the physician occasionally suppresses TSH production by giving thyroid-replacement medication in order to prevent further growth of the thyroid. It is rare for a depressed TSH value to be caused by a disruption in hypophyseal function. In patients where this is the case there is, in contrast to all other states involving a lack of TSH, a simultaneous thyroid hypofunction.

We should also mention that in cases with only slightly decreased TSH measurements, the physician can conduct a thyrotropin-releasing hormone test (TRH test) in order to diagnose early stages of thyroid hyperfunction. In this test, the patient is given TRH (thyrotropin-releasing hormone), which in healthy people stimulates TSH production, but has no effect in patients with hyperthyroidism.

►► *Thyroxin*

Other names: Tetraiodothyronine
Abbreviation: T4
Description: T4 is a thyroid hormone that stimulates the metabolism and maturation of nearly all of our body cells. It contains four iodine atoms per molecule (hence the name tetraiodothyronine, from the

Greek *tetra:* four), of which one is removed in the liver or kidney, leading to the formation of the metabolically much more active T3 (triiodothyronine). T3 and T4 are for the most part bound to carrier proteins, and are thereby rendered inert. Only the unbound portions (0.3% of T3 and T4) are active hormones. These portions are designated free T4 (FT4) and free T3 (FT3). The normal concentration of T3 is significantly lower than that of T4.

Units (factor): μg/dl, nmol/l (12.87 for T4)

Normal range: T4: 5.5–12.5 μg/dl, FT4: 0.9–2.3 ng/dl, T3: 80–200 ng/dl, FT3: 0.25–0.60 ng/dl

Medical significance: The above tests are used in combination with other thyroid tests to determine if patients are euthyroid (normal), or have developed hyper- or hypothyroidism. Elevated values may indicate hyperthyroidism, while decreased values may indicate hypothyroidism. With thyroid hyperfunction, patients develop insomnia, diarrhea, hair loss, tremors, and weight loss, while hypofunction leads to depression, fatigue, and weight gain.

►► *Triglycerides*

Other names: triacylglycerol

Abbreviation: TG

Description: Triglycerides are our body's main fuel. They are synthesized in the liver from fat and sugar in the diet, and are stored mainly in fatty tissue. When necessary, these fats are consumed as an energy source in the muscles and in other organs. Triglycerides are transported in the bloodstream. Since fats are not water-soluble, triglycerides can be transported only in "packaged" form, mainly in the very low density lipoproteins (VLDL).

Units (factor): mg/dl, mmol/l (0.0113)

Reference interval (normal range): Triglyceride levels depend mainly on fat reserves and, to a lesser extent, on age. Thus, normal ranges differ widely among populations. More important than the normal range is the consensus-value of 200 mg/dl. This value should not be exceeded, in order to avoid arteriosclerotic disease. The lower limit of triglyceride concentrations is approximately 10 mg/dl.

Medical significance: Increased values are found mainly in overweight patients as a result of increased body fat reserves. Elevated values may also be seen in people suffering from diabetes. In both, there is a disruption in the absorption of blood fat into fat cells, as regulated by the hormone insulin. More rarely, high concentrations of TG may be due to an inflammation of the liver or pancreas. In children, a congenital fat metabolism disorder may be the etiology. Decreased values can be found in patients with malnutrition and hyperthyroidism.

▶▶ *Triiodothyronine (T3)*—See Thyroxin

▶▶ *Urea*

Abbreviation: BUN
Description: Urea is a catabolic product of our protein metabolism, which is excreted by the kidneys, similiar to uric acid.
Units (factor): mg/dl, mmol/l (0.357)
Normal range: 8–23 mg/dl, increasing with age
Medical significance: Elevated levels of urea, as with creatinine, indicate a reduction in kidney function. Reduced concentrations are found in patients suffering from a decrease in dietary protein, in those with an extremely small amount of muscle mass, and during pregnancy.

▶▶ *Uric Acid*

Description: Uric acid is a metabolite which is formed mainly when substances in the cells' nuclei are broken down (nucleic acids), and which is secreted via the kidneys into the urine.
Units (factor): mg/dl, mmol/l (0.0595)
Normal range: Females: 2.7–7.3 mg/dl; Males: 4–8.5 mg/dl.
Medical significance: Increased uric acid concentration in the blood is diagnostically important. It mainly indicates the genetic metabolic disease, gout, in which secretion of uric acid through the kidneys is decreased. Men are affected by this disease seven times more often than women. The most typical symptom is a painful inflammation of the big toe's large joint, but other joints can also be affected.

Other reasons for increased levels of uric acid are diseases of the kidneys or the blood, as well as various medications that interfere with the secretion of uric acid. Some medications also cause a decrease in uric acid concentration in the blood that has no negative effect on the patient.

INDEX

ILLUSTRATION CREDITS

Photos of blood sampling techniques (pp. 22 and 24) are by Klaus Krischok, München. © 1991 BLV.

Photo of the Blood Bank Centrifuge (p. 26) courtesy of Jouan, Inc. © 1992 Jouan, Inc.

Photo of the 480 Clinical Flame Photometer (p. 31) courtesy of Ciba Corning Diagnostics Limited, UK. © 1992 Ciba Corning Diagnostics Ltd., UK.

Photo of the Kodak Ektachem 700XR Analyzer C (p. 34) courtesy of Kodak Canada, Inc., Clinical Products. © 1992 Kodak Canada, Inc.

Photo of the ONE TOUCH® II Blood Glucose Meter (p. 36) courtesy of LifeScan Canada Ltd., a Johnson and Johnson Co. © 1992 LifeScan Canada Ltd.

Diagrams on pp. 4, 23, 147 from Barbara von Damnitz, Grünwald. Diagrams on pp. 87, 88, 135 from Gertraud Bosch, Die Hauswirtschaft, Band Gesundheitspflege, BLV München, 3, Auflage 1989. Diagram on p. 108 from Dr. med. Ulf Nicolausson, Das praktische Gesundheitsbuch für die Familie, BLV, München, 1984. Diagram on p. 125 from Lehrmittelverlag Wilhelm Hagemann, Düsseldorf (Lehrtafeln der Reihe "Körper des Menschen"). All © 1991 BLV, München.

Information for pp. 7, 8, 34 from Prof. Dr. med. Peter Mathes, Ratgeber Herzinfarkt, BLV, München, 1991.